To D
warm regards
Ricardo
16/6/23

DARE TO DIFFER

Compliments from

[signature]
8/6/93

DARE TO DIFFER

A DOCTOR'S QUEST FOR A GENTLE CURE

Dr Kusum S. Chand

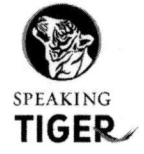

SPEAKING TIGER

SPEAKING TIGER BOOKS LLP
125A, Ground Floor, Shahpur Jat, near Asiad Village,
New Delhi 110049

First published by Speaking Tiger Books 2022

Copyright © Dr Kusum S. Chand 2022

ISBN: 978-93-5447-329-6
eISBN: 978-93-5447-330-2

10 9 8 7 6 5 4 3 2 1

Typeset in Minion Pro by SÜRYA, New Delhi
Printed at Chaman Enterprises, New Delhi

All rights reserved.
No part of this publication may be reproduced, transmitted,
or stored in a retrieval system, in any form or by any means, electronic,
mechanical, photocopying, recording or otherwise,
without the prior permission of the publisher.

This book is sold subject to the condition that it shall not,
by way of trade or otherwise, be lent, resold, hired out,
or otherwise circulated, without the publisher's prior
consent, in any form of binding or cover other
than that in which it is published.

CONTENTS

A Note from the Author — vii
Foreword — ix
Introduction — xiii
Dictionary of Medical Terms — xv
Abbreviations: Homeopathy — xxiii

Prologue — 1

PART ONE: TRYST WITH HOMEOPATHY AS AN ALLOPATH

1. Road to Becoming a Medical Doctor — 7
2. Disillusionment Starts — 11
3. Encounter with a Homeopath — 15
4. Homeopathy Excites Interest — 21
5. Learning Homeopathy — 26
6. Ups and Downs In Practice — 33
7. Dilemma: To Be or Not To Be — 46

PART TWO: TRYST WITH HOMEOPATHY AS A HOMEOPATH

8. Decision to Restrict Medical Practice to Homeopathy — 57
9. Of Challenges and Learnings — 59
10. Setting My Own Pattern — 62
11. Experiments and Experiences — 65

PART THREE: EXPERIMENTS IN CHILDHOOD DISEASES

12. Homeopathy for Children: My Thoughts   81
13. Childhood Diseases' Case Studies   83

PART FOUR: EXPERIMENTS IN URINARY COMPLAINTS

14. Integration of Two Systems for Urinary Complaints   101
15. Management of Urinary Complaints   105

PART FIVE: EXPERIMENTS IN THE FIELD OF TUBERCULOSIS

16. Background   115
17. The Project: Role of Homeopathy In Tuberculosis   121
18. Outcome of the Project   124
19. Idea of Formation of a Homeopathic Regime   134
20. Experiences In a Hospital Setting   139

PART SIX: THE WAY FORWARD

21. Immunity, Disease and Medicine   159
22. My Dream   164
23. In Conclusion   167

Acknowledgements   170
Appendix: Case Histories of Tuberculosis   172
References   212

A Note from the Author

This book has been written because a story had to be told. Writing a book seemed to be an easier way of sharing my stories about two medical treatments and answering the *whys* and *hows* I have been asked so many times. And it had to be written by me. Someone else may have got it all wrong.

Popularity and success notwithstanding, I have wrestled for years with the intricacies and complexities of straddling two streams of medicine. I am a proud product of modern medicine (allopathy); a postgraduate of the latter half of the twentieth century, an era when modern medicine was growing by leaps and bounds. However, my unprejudiced mind could discern a weakness in the therapeutic system and so, instead of basking in its success, I embarked on decades of more learning and experimentation with homeopathy, a system much ridiculed, yet, surviving for more than two centuries. It took me more than two decades to personally validate its effectiveness, a period when I became popular as a 'two prescriptions doctor'. I learnt that allopathy and homeopathy are like two colours of the spectrum, blue and yellow, good by themselves. But when they come together, a new colour—green—is formed, which denotes good health and wellness.

In formulating each prescription, my main concern has been the health and wellness of the patient and preserving my integrity as a doctor.

This book is full of case histories. While all the cases are factual, names have been changed to protect the privacy of the patients. The first part should make for an enjoyable read for the uninitiated; the non-believer in complementary medicine and the lay person. The second part is more medical, albeit written in a manner that while a homeopath and/or a medical student may benefit from it, any lay reader will also find it an interesting read. The subsequent part, dealing with disease-wise case histories, has been documented keeping in mind medical practitioners. The last part, 'The Way Forward', is my vision of an integrated medical practice, a must read for all interested in public health.

Dear Reader, the effort has been to not ask questions or to give answers, but to share with you my confusion, disillusionment, excitement and eureka moments. This book does not fall neatly into any one category. And thereby hangs a tale which I hope you will enjoy.

Foreword

The book *Dare to Differ* by Dr Kusum Chand, brings to light the serious threat of antibiotic resistance that the world has been grappling with and how integrating homeopathy with allopathy can be the most innovative and inexpensive strategy in the treatment of intractable infections. A World Health Organization (WHO) survey carried out across 22 high- and low-income countries between March 2016 to July 2017 linked antibiotic resistance to several serious bacterial infections and raised many red flags among health professionals, who admitted that it is one of the biggest threats to global public health. According to the Center of Disease Control and Prevention's (CDC's) 2019 Antibiotic Resistance (AR) Threats Report, more than 35,000 people die every year in the USA due to the failing effect of antibiotics.

Dr Chand's first encounter with homeopathy was when she suffered from a recurrent urinary tract infection due to a drug-resistant strain of bacteria. After much reluctance, she finally tried homeopathy and was both amazed and intrigued by the results. Her curiosity ignited, she joined Nehru Homeopathic Medical College and Hospital, the top medical school of homeopathy, in 1983 as a visiting professor to teach and interact with students, residents and experienced teachers. Since I was working as the Senior Resident in the hospital, I used to interact with her for learning clinical medicine and making a correct diagnosis of the admitted patients.

She gained popularity as the 'two prescriptions doctor' while practising as a general physician at Delhi's Masonic Polyclinic, when she gave her patients the best of both worlds using both allopathic and homeopathic medicines. As time passed, she received tremendous acknowledgement for her homeopathic prescriptions. This motivated her to be different and bring a difference. She left the conventional path and switched to homeopathy completely. Breaking from the elite ranks of a conventional doctor was not easy, yet she not only left it but also acquired the Member of Faculty of Homeopathy (MF Hom), a Master's degree in homeopathy, from the Royal London College of Faculty of Homeopathy, United Kingdom. This empowered her legally to prescribe homeopathy to her patients in India.

Her grit to help the patients and society through her knowledge knew no bounds. Throughout her journey, she examined homeopathy with a critical eye and challenged the classical system. She kept experimenting with multiple medicines, frequent repetitions, frequent change of medicine, dosage and mode of dispensing. She is a strong votary of bringing change in the practice of homeopathy, and has often expressed the view that the great discoveries that do not adapt to altered situations die. She believes that if the world changes and we do not, we become of no use to the world. Our principles cease being principles and just ossify. The change is not to forget our principles, but to fulfil them, not to lose our identity but to keep our relevance. It is important to develop in ways that better reflects the altered situation around us. She dared to approach patients in a different manner only for their benefit. As mentioned in the book, she encountered innumerable chronic and acute cases that were treated in no time.

In 1999, the Government of Delhi decided to undertake a research project in evaluating homeopathy in multidrug-resistant tuberculosis. I approached Dr Kusum Chand for this project as she had the unique distinction of having conventional as well as homeopathic qualifications. She readily agreed to join the project and worked with all her might for its success. She was the lead consultant for the project and the journey was very educative. For the first time any such experiment was being conducted wherein conventional medicine as well as homeopathy was being used concurrently in a disease having immense public health importance. Several observational, along with one double-blind randomized control trial, were undertaken over a period of one decade. Dr Chand has described the outcome of these studies very carefully in this book, which can motivate and inspire others to follow and do further research in this area.

The journey of Dr Chand till the publication of this book has been immensely gratifying for the profession. The book not only shares her involvement with two completely opposite systems of medicine, but also discusses the challenges she faced during her transition to homeopathy and how she bravely overcame them.

Peter Gotzsche, co-founder of the reputed Cochrane collaboration, estimated that prescribed medication is the third most common cause of death globally after heart disease and cancer (*The Guardian*, 30 August 2018). If homeopathy is to thrive, it needs to address criticisms, become more professional, sharper and facing outwards, so that it can continue to offer and secure its contribution to curing diseases and enhancing health and wellness. The contribution of Dr Chand in the form of this book is very important information for integrating homeopathy in the public health domain.

I would like to recommend this book to everyone who dares to be different and takes up challenges in life. It is recommended to the patients who get ridiculed for opting for homeopathy as a system of choice: this will give them the confidence to use homeopathy not only in difficult situations but also as a first line of choice for day-to-day problems. This book is also meant for the homeopathic doctors who wish to take up challenging cases and can find their paths based on the various treatment strategies shared by the author. They are also encouraged to develop their own successful treatment regimens and share with the profession instead of getting bogged down by the pressure of practising on dotted lines.

It is meant for allopathic practitioners who look down on homeopathy and refrain from integrating it for the benefit of patients. The idea of this book is to promote an integrated system of medicine with a goal to cure and relieve the patients of their sickness in a holistic way.

Dr Raj K. Manchanda

Director
Directorate of AYUSH,
Government of Delhi
Former Director General,
Central Council for Research in Homeopathy,
Government of India
Secretary, for Information and Communication,
Liga Medicorum Homeopathica

Introduction

In Europe and the USA, integrated (or integrative) medicine is very popular. Integrated medicine is loosely defined as combining the best of both conventional and complementary and traditional medicine systems. Whilst many agree with these lofty aims, looking more closely under the surface of 'integrated medicine' reveals that it is more often 'pluralistic', rather than 'integrated', medicine: a single patient being treated in parallel by conventional and complementary medicine practitioners, with each operating in their own silos. 'Integration' implies that the total is more than the sum of the parts, but often we see that despite 'talking the talk', integrated medicine is often, at best, only 'the sum of the parts'. By contrast, *Dare to Differ* does not only 'talk the talk', it 'walks the walk'. Dr Kusum Chand describes her fascinating walk through life, first as a conventional doctor, then as a homeopathic doctor, but most of all as an immensely caring person with a scientific mindset.

Her book is both easy to read and informative, both personal and factual. As the title suggests, her 'courage to be different' is commendable, and inspired by her quest to find a gentle cure for her patients. In this quest, she is not guided by homeopathic, nor conventional, dogma. She consistently applies the scientific spirit of 'putting things to the test', a spirit which also guided Hahnemann in his discovery of homeopathy.

In doing so, she is truly exploring the essence of integrated medicine: instead of polarizing conventional medicine and homeopathy, she, for instance, looks for ways in which homeopathic medicines can help make conventional antibiotics work better. Her work and experience in the domain of anti-microbial resistance (AMR) is invaluable. Apart from being a major problem already, AMR is set to become one of the greatest medical challenges the world will face in the coming decades.

Despite increasing support worldwide for the concepts and ideals of 'integrated medicine', a lot of work still needs to be done on different ways and models in which conventional medicine and homeopathy can be integrated. I wholeheartedly recommend Dr Chand's book as a source of inspiration and guidance on this path.

Dr Robbert van Haselen
Director, World Integrated Medicine Forum
Director, International Institute for
Integrated Medicine (INTMEDI)

Dictionary of Medical Terms

AFB	Acid Fast Bacillus
Akt4	follow-up comprises *R-Cinex* 600 mg od, *Mycobutol* 100 mg od, *Pyzina* 750 mg, *Benadon* 40 mg½ od
Amikacin®	antibiotic
Amoxycillin	antibiotic
Ampicillin®	antibiotic
analgesic nephropathy	deterioration of kidney function from the intake of pain-relieving drugs
antibiotic	a drug which destroys bacteria by killing it or preventing its multiplication
ATT	Anti-tubercular Treatment
Augmentin duo®	combination of two antibiotics
auxillary treatment	any therapy that increases a primary treatment's efficacy
Bifilac®	helps in restoring the normal microbial flora of the intestine
blinding process	method adopted in a research project where the patient does not know what medicine he/she

	is getting and the prescriber does not know what he/she is prescribing
Burkholderia cepacia	a type of bacteria
capreomycin or kanamycin	injectable broad-spectrum antibiotic
Cat III	one of the regimes of ATT
Cefixime®	cephalosporin antibiotic
chest auscultation	hearing sounds in the chest through a stethoscope
chronic disease	lasts/recurs for more than three months
Citrobacter koseri	a type of bacteria
colic	waxing and waning pain in the abdomen
constitutional medicine	the homeopathic thought behind constitutional medicine is that if a medicine is chosen, encompassing all the symptoms of the disease and the patient's reactions to the environment and people, eating and sleeping habits, food preferences, that medicine will remove the underlying disease along with the symptoms
DST	Drug-sensitivity test
dyscrasia	a premorbid condition, state of imbalance, with a propensity to develop diseases like tuberculosis, cancer
dyspepsia	indigestion
dyspnoea	breathlessness

E. coli	specific type of bacteria, common cause of urinary tract infection
E.B. Nash	American homeopath
empirically	reliance on information obtained through observation, experiment, or experience
eructation	release of air or gas from the stomach or esophagus through the mouth
expectoration	discharge of matter from the throat or lungs by coughing or hawking and spitting
exploratory laparotomy	surgical opening of abdomen to find the cause of disease
extremities	limbs or appendages of the body, particularly the hands and feet
flatulence	the accumulation of gas in the alimentary canal
FNAC	Fine Needle Aspiration Cytology
Hahnemann	a German physician, Christian Friedrich Samuel Hahnemann (1755–1843), is the founder of homeopathy. When Hahnemann first named the discipline in 1807, mainstream medicine involved ineffective practices such as bloodletting and purging. Complex mixtures such as Venice treacle which comprised 64 substances including opium, myrrh and even viper's flesh was also being used. He developed the basic

	principles of homeopathy while translating a medical paper by William Cullen into German. Cullen had written that eating cinchona bark could cure malaria, which led Hahnemann to ingest some of the bark and investigate its effects. Hahnemann developed symptoms similar to those seen in malaria such as fever, joint pain and chills. He then began to promote the 'law of similars'. His methodical dilution and succussion technique of preparing the medicine, which he called remedy, made the similia principle usable in disease with minimum aggravation.
hepatitis	inflammation of the liver
homeothermic	having a relatively uniform body temperature maintained nearly independent of the environmental temperature
Klebsiella	a type of bacteria
lymph node	a small bean-shaped structure that is part of the body's immune system
lymphadenitis (adenopathy)	inflammation of lymph node, caseating necrosis cheesy dead tissue
macrophage	a key component of the innate immune system that resides in

Dictionary of Medical Terms xix

	tissues, where it functions as an immune sentinel
marasmus	a type of protein-energy malnutrition that can affect anyone but is mainly seen in children.
maxillary sinusitis	inflammation of paranasal maxillary sinus, situated in the cheekbone
MDR TB	Multidrug-resistant Tuberculosis
non-Hodgkin's lymphoma	a type of cancer that begins in the lymphatic system, which is part of the body's germ-fighting immune system
olfaction	through smell
palpable	which can be felt by touch
paroxysmal	symptom recurs in sudden fits/attacks
pathogenicity	the property of causing disease
Pharmacopeia	a book describing drugs, chemicals and medicinal preparations, especially one issued by an officially recognized authority and serving as a standard
pleural involvement	involvement of the covering of the lung
pneumonitis	inflammation of the lung
potency (in homeopathy)	the number of times a remedy has been diluted and succussed, taken as a measure of the strength of the effect it will produce

potentization	a process in which a substance is diluted with alcohol or distilled water and then vigorously shaken in a process called 'succussion'
Professor Hugo	Hugo von Mohl (8 April 1805– 1 April 1872) was a German botanist from Stuttgart
pruritis	itching
pyelography	X-ray of the kidney
Repertory	a compilation of symptoms as elicited in a person; the same symptom could be produced by many medicines, but in different intensity
retrosternal	behind the sternum, also called the breastbone
rubric	a symptom expressed in *Repertory* as rubric
SDM	self-defence mechanism
Serratia maracescens	a type of bacteria
similimum	a remedy selected because it causes symptoms similar to those that the practitioner wishes to treat
Staphylococcus aureus	bacteria causing many types of infections
Streptococcus haemolyticus	bacteria causing throat infections, scarlet fever etc.
syndromic	different diseases present with same set of signs and symptoms, particularly in young children; a holistic and integrated approach

	to treatment is a syndromic approach
synthetic analogue	chemically prepared, similar in action
Taylor's brace	(short/long type) is a lightweight spinal brace, supports and immobilizes the spine in a neutral position, still permitting the requisite body movement
trigeminal neuralgia	also known as tic douloureux, is a distinctive facial pain syndrome that may become recurrent and chronic.
Trinorm®	capsule that treats and prevents urinary infections

Assessment criteria of Indian National Tuberculosis Control Programme, revised (RNTCP)

i. *Cure:* a patient who has completed treatment and has been consistently culture negative (with at least 5 consecutive negative results in the last 12 to 15 months). If one culture positive is reported during the last three quarters, the patient will be considered cured provided it is followed by three consecutive negative cultures, taken at least 30 days apart, provided there is clinical evidence of improvement.

ii. *Treatment failure:* treatment will be considered to have failed if two or more of the five cultures recorded in the final 12–15 months are positive or if any of the three final are culture positive.

iii. *Defaulter:* a patient whose treatment was interrupted for two or more consecutive months for any reasons. In this study, patients who did not complete treatment for 24 months were considered as defaulters.

iv. *Time to culture conversion:* duration from initiation of treatment to the date of first of the two consecutive negative cultures, taken at least one month apart, irrespective of the subsequent results.

B	basophil
c/o	complaints of current disease
DLC	differential leucocytic count
E	eosin
ESR	Erythrocytic Sedimentation Rate
h/o	history of all previous/existing ailments besides current disease
Hb	haemoglobin, total leucocytic count (TLC)
L	lymphocyte
P	polymorph/neutrophil

Abbreviations: Homeopathy

All-c.	Allium cepa
Ant-c.	Antimonium crudum
Ant-t.	Antimonium tartaricum
Arn.	Arnica montana
Ars.	Arsenicum album
Ars-i.	Arsenicun iodatum
Bac.	Bacillinum
Bar-c.	Baryta carbonica
Bell.	Belladonna
Berb.	Berberis vulgaris
Borx.	Borax veneta
Bry.	Bryonia alba
Calc.	Calcarea carbonica
Calc-f.	Calcarea fluorica
Calc-i.	Calcarea iodata
Calc-p.	Calcarea phosphorica
Calen.	Calendula officinalis
Canth.	Cantharis vesicatoria
Carb-v.	Carbo vegetabilis
Cina.	Cina maritima

Cist.	Cistus canadensis
Clem.	Clematis erecta
Cocc.	Cocculus indicus
Colch.	Colchicum autumnale
Coloc.	Colocynthis
Dol.	Dolichos pruriens
Ferr-p.	Ferrum phosphoricum
Graph.	Graphites
Ham.	Hamamelis virginica
Hep.	Hepar sulphuris
Ign.	Ignatia amara
Ip.	Ipecacuanha
Kali-bi.	Kalium bichromicum
Kali-c.	Kalium carbonicum
Kali-i.	Kalium iodatum
Lach.	Lachesis mutus
Led.	Ledum palustre
Lyc.	Lycopodium clavatum
Mag-c.	Magnesium carbonicum
Mag-p.	Magnesium phosphoricum
Merc-c.	Mercurius corrosivus
Merc-i-r.	Mercurius iodatus ruber
Nat-m.	Natrum muriaticum
Nat-p.	Natrum phosphoricum
Nux-v.	Nux vomica
Phos.	Phosphorus
Phyt.	Phytolacca decandra

Psor.	Psorinum
Puls.	Pulsatilla pratensis
R87	Homeopathic patent medicine
Rhus-t.	Rhus toxicodendron
Sang.	Sanguinaria canadensis
Sep.	Sepia officinalis
Sil.	Silicea terra
Spong.	Spongia tosta
Staph.	Staphysagria
Staph.	Staphysagria
Staphycoc.	Staphylococcinum
Sulph.	Sulphur
Symph.	Symphytum officinale
Thuj.	Thuja occidentalis
Thuj.	Thuja occidentalis
Tub.	Tuberculinum bovinum Kent
Urt-u.	Urtica urens
Verb.	Verbascum thapsus

Prologue

Ignoring the NO VISITORS sign, I entered the microbiology laboratory, secure in the knowledge I could do so, as I had recently finished a few months of training in the department. The hand holding the drug-sensitivity plate shook slightly as I checked and rechecked the laboratory number, wishing that it was not the number that I had gone to check first thing in the morning before starting the daily routine at the hospital, but it was THE number. The round specks on the upside of the plate were staring at me. These specks were indicative of the growth of a bacterium, which had grown in spite of all the antibiotic discs present in the culture medium. The bacterium by the name *Staphylococcus aureus* was defying me, laughing at me—it seemed to be saying 'treat me, if you can.' Its growth was an indication that it was resistant to all available antibiotics. I was crestfallen, all the complications of a drug-resistant urinary tract infection flashed in my mind. But my confidence and faith in modern medicine soon perked me up. Science was making rapid progress in every field, new drugs were being discovered every other day. I was confident that soon an appropriate antibiotic would be found for this bug; till then, all that was required of me was to take precautions and keep a check on the infection. However, the frequent urine examinations and yearly intravenous pyelographs created the fear of having an incurable disease. I would get a test done because of burning pain during urination, but the test report would be normal. I was increasingly becoming a nervous wreck. All I wished for was something that would relieve the nagging symptoms and give peace to my mind.

As luck would have it, a gentleman in my husband's office practised homeopathy as a hobby. My husband asked him if homeopathy had something for my condition. 'Yes,' was the prompt and confident reply. I was reluctant to meet him because, in my mind, homeopathy was only good for skin problems and vague psychological symptoms; not for serious infections like mine. On the husband's insistence, I decided to give homeopathy a try. After a few months, grudgingly, I had to admit a reduction in the frequency of symptoms and urine examinations. I was, however, still not convinced about homeopathy being a scientific method of treatment. When I told the gentleman this, he smiled and told me a story.

The story was about two fellow scientists with the drug, belladonna, at the centre of it. *Atropa belladonna*, commonly known as belladonna or deadly nightshade, is a poisonous perennial herbaceous plant. It contains chemicals that can be toxic, leading to a dry mouth, enlarged pupils, blurred vision, dry red skin, fever, fast heartbeat, inability to urinate or sweat, hallucinations, spasms, mental problems, convulsions, coma, you name it.

One scientist, wanting to find out the active principle that caused the symptoms, analyses the plant in the laboratory. He identifies the active principle as 'atropine', studies its action on animals and records all the details. He realizes that it acts by stimulating the autonomic nervous system and catalogues the medical conditions where it can be used. For example, its action on the eyes can be useful in the examination of the retina; action on the heart can be useful in patients with slow heart rate; action on skin can be useful in patients who suffer from excessive sweating, and so on. The associated symptoms, besides the action desired in a particular disease, are named side-effects of the drug. He further works on this chemical, producing its synthetic analogue; modifying it in various ways, either to reduce the side-effects or to change the duration of action in order to maximize its use with minimum unwanted effects. This is science, the foundation of modern medicine or allopathy.

The other scientist studies many cases of belladonna poisoning and catalogues the entire range of symptoms. He realizes people react with different intensity to the same exposure: from bright shiny eyes with a slight flush on the face to a delirious state, but observes that some symptoms are present in all the cases. Then he gives a minute dose of the belladonna extract to the delirious patient with bright shiny eyes, flushed face and history of being exposed to belladonna. He finds the symptoms disappear, and the patient is normal in no time. He gives the same belladonna extract to patients with the same symptoms but who are unexposed to belladonna. There also the symptoms are removed, making the patient feel comfortable and normal. At the same time, he notices an initial aggravation in the symptoms before they disappear; in some patients this aggravation is marked. He feels that the aggravation could be due to more quantity of the medicine. So, he experiments in a methodical manner, reducing the dose mathematically and recording it meticulously, till the symptoms of the disease disappear without perceptible aggravation. In this way, he reaches an effective dose which has an incredibly minute quantity of medicine. This is homeopathy.

The homeopath said as he came to the end of the story, 'Homeopathy is also a science.'

The story impacted me. A scientific mind is an admission that we do not know everything. That there are new discoveries possible, based on new observations, which in turn will lead to continuously changing our beliefs. I was also a scientist and curious about new discoveries and willing to change my mind because of it. The seed of homeopathy was sown.

The following pages describe my tryst with homeopathy, first as an allopath general practitioner. And then as a specialist homeopath with a background of allopathy.

PART ONE

Tryst with Homeopathy as an Allopath

One

Road to Becoming a Medical Doctor

My father came from a feudalistic background, where educating girls beyond a certain point was considered to be wasteful expenditure. He himself was a graduate of Delhi's St. Stephen's College, a co-ed institution at that time, and was married to the sister of his friend and batchmate. Both my parents believed in modern education and put me in an English-medium school, against the wishes of my paternal grandfather, who controlled the affairs of the family with an iron fist. My mother was keen on my becoming a doctor and my father acquiesced to this wish. In the eighth standard I was enrolled in Lady Irwin School, which had the best science laboratories in Delhi, particularly its biology laboratory. I vividly remember my first day in the bio-lab. To study the skeletal system, each one of us was given a frog. The strong odour emitted during this process affected me and, unable to tolerate it, I went to my father and asked if biology could be exchanged for mechanical drawing. He refused point-blank, saying that girls don't become engineers (this was the year 1955). His words, 'It's fine if you are not up for this. After you complete high school, you will be married off,' were enough of a threat for me to bear the smells in the biology laboratory. However, subsequent experiments on frogs were exciting, and I soon started excelling in them.

In the summer of 1958, my father enrolled me for a pre-medical course. His family suggested a matrimonial match for me, which was successfully warded off on the grounds of my being too young for marriage and the boy in question being too short in height. The following year, I got admission in both of Delhi's medical colleges: Lady Hardinge Medical College and Maulana Azad Medical College. The former was a well-established institution and had the unique distinction of being the only medical college in India that exclusively trained women undergraduate students. It was attached to a hospital for women and children. The latter was new, but attached to a big multispeciality hospital, Irwin Hospital [now known as Lok Nayak Jai Prakash Narayan Hospital (LNJP)]. My father was keen on Lady Hardinge Medical College, while I felt that confining my education to the fields of gynaecology and paediatrics would mean an incomplete education. At that time there were very few women physicians in India, and most were in the field of gynaecology or paediatrics, while I wanted to be a general physician. After a week of a tussle, my mother agreed to take my side, albeit with many conditions attached: I was to come back home straight from college (in my first year of college, she would be at the gates of our house, sharp at five in the evening every day, waiting for me); no boyfriends; marriage only with the man of my parents' choice, etc. I agreed to all the conditions and enrolled in the college of my choice: Maulana Azad Medical College.

Out of the twelve subjects taught in the five-year course, my favourites were anatomy (I loved doing dissection of the human body); pathology and microbiology (study of cause and effect of a disease and its healing process); and clinical medicine (using symptoms to find out what is happening inside the body through inductive reasoning).

My grandfather fell sick when I was in my third year and had started clinical training in a hospital. As a doctor-in-the-making, I looked after him, and very soon he was on his feet again. He was so thankful for having an in-house doctor, and impressed by the treatment, that he spoke the scriptchanging words, 'Let the girl complete her studies.' This, coming from my grandfather, was enough to put an end to any talk of marriage till the end of my graduation.

Once I graduated, it was time to think about the future. My parents actively started looking for a suitable match for me and I started actively thinking about specialization. One night, while on duty in the surgical ward, I got talking to a senior who had recently done her postgraduation in surgery. She was finding it difficult to get a 'suitable' match, someone who was equally educated and would have no objection to her working in a hospital. Having studied so hard and for so long, she felt it would be very disappointing to settle for less. The next morning saw me convinced that pursing a non-clinical specialization would be better for me in the long run, though I was very fond of medicine as a subject and had enjoyed my stint in surgery and been appreciated by the seniors.

I worked in the microbiology department, on a temporary post, for a few months. As a permanent post was not available, and I didn't want to start postgraduation before marriage, I joined the anatomy department—another favourite non-clinical subject—of Maulana Azad Medical College in Delhi.

In the meantime, my father had found a suitable match, suggested by his close friend. The boy in question, Satish

Chand, was a non-medico; he was from the Indian Railway Service, posted at Bhavnagar, Gujarat, Western Railway division. Till then, my parents were looking for a medico, as it was felt that my education would not go to waste, if both husband and wife had the same profession. My family was attracted by the alliance, because of a similar family background and the boy had an impressive personality and was broadminded in his outlook. He had no objection to my practising medicine. The evening this proposal was revealed to me, I was going to hospital for night duty. That night, the hospital grapevine revealed a major fight between a working doctor-couple. That set me thinking that being in the same profession did not assure marital harmony, which I was hoping to achieve by marrying a medico, more than the desire to practise medicine. In subsequent meetings, Satish voiced a concern that if after marriage we could not live together, then there seemed to be no point of marriage. At that time, he was posted in Ajmer, but was trying to get a transfer to Delhi, our hometown. He said that if that happened, then he would leave his job and start his own business. This seemed logical to me; so, after the engagement ceremony, I went with my resignation letter to the head of the department. He was a kind, wise man and felt that it was foolhardy of me to give up a permanent job. He advised me against doing so and generously offered to sanction as many leaves as I may need. But I was set on resigning and did so, though for some time this decision appeared to be really foolish as, after marriage, I was in Ajmer for barely three weeks when my husband got his transfer orders to Delhi.

After six months, I enrolled in Delhi University for postgraduation in medicine. Possibly the hand of destiny was guiding me in all this. I was destined to be a clinician.

Two

Disillusionment Starts

The day I received my postgraduate degree in medicine, in the year 1970, I was on top of the world. I felt that I knew all there was to know about diseases and their cures. Everything was scientific. Infectious diseases like typhoid, malaria, meningitis, cholera, pneumonia, scarlet fever had been won over; the causative organism, the microbe was known. It could be seen under a microscope and cultured in a laboratory. The specific antibiotic against the microbe had been studied thoroughly in its mode and duration of action and a safe dosage had been ascertained through animal experiments. Smallpox was almost eradicated, heart transplants were successful, human longevity had increased, infant mortality decreased. Having worked in a large hospital like LNJP, treating 'n' number of serious, end-stage patients, I felt that allopathy was the best system of medicine.

By this time, my husband had found an alternate vocation in business and was contemplating leaving his existing government job. My maternal uncle was in construction business in Assam and his maternal uncle had property in Delhi; both jointly formed a construction company and made him the active working partner. It was also time for us to think about starting a family. So, instead of taking up a job, I took a sabbatical from medicine. But job or no job, a doctor can never be without patients. In no time, I was the 'easily available' first-line doctor for family and friends. My prescriptions, apart from being free, must have been effective for people to keep coming back to me. So much so that in our joint family, everything pertaining to medicine fell on me.

A child in the family had a respiratory allergy. Three senior paediatricians were looking after him. One was an allergy specialist who would recommend steam inhalations three times a day, through a pipe made by rolling newspaper. Another would prescribe an antibiotic, which was negated by the third who felt it adversely affected development of bones. All this was confusing and frustrating as the child still continued to suffer. The family was consoled by the assurance that the allergy would disappear as he grew older. Seeing all this, my confidence in medicine was shaken.

This was also the period when I was troubled by a recurrent urinary tract infection. The episodes in the beginning were few and far between, and a few days of antibiotics were enough to cure them. Gradually, these became more frequent and needed a longer course of antibiotics. This was in spite of precautions such as adequate water intake, dietary restrictions, proper emptying of bladder and regular urinary tests. One day, the urine culture report showed the growth of a bacterium, which was resistant to all available antibiotics. This set me thinking that maybe the current knowledge of medicine was lacking in something that prevented the complete annihilation of a disease. When confronted with this drug-resistant infection, I felt defeated and crestfallen.

Subsequently, in the year 1974, I joined Masonic Clinic as an honorary consultant physician. It was a newly opened facility and close to my house, which suited me as I could both remain in touch with my profession and take care of my family. The clinic had started with a pathology laboratory, with a few doctors also available for consultation. However, the doctors would come only if patients were waiting, while patients wanted the surety of a doctor's presence. Hence, though the laboratory was doing well, the medical centre had not taken off. I was very regular, always present in the clinic for the entire duration of the stipulated time and was diligent with patients. Once a patient came, complaining of pain in his knees, alongside headache and lethargy, since some months. He said that the pain would be slightly better when he took pain-relieving drugs, but would come back when he stopped taking the painkillers. Detailed examination showed that his blood pressure was high. I treated him for hypertension and, as his blood pressure came down, his knee pain vanished.

Attendance was good on the days I was on duty at the clinic, and when the secretary asked the other consultants why the attendance was poor on their days, the reply was that patients came because I was a young, good-looking, female doctor, conveniently ignoring my regularity, diligence and competence. Soon the clinic became popular for its laboratory and medical care. This reached the ears of my Professor of Medicine, Dr Hari Vaishnav, who called me and complimented me, saying that it felt nice when his students did good work.

Masonic was an outpatient clinic. I was treating cases of fever, cold, cough and early stage diabetes, hypertension and so on. Patients often complained of troublesome symptoms, even after proper diagnosis and treatment. The disease would be at the functional level, without any structural changes in the tissues. One wished for the milder protocol of a gentler medicine as an effective form of treatment which would stimulate the natural ability of the organism to heal itself. Gradually the euphoria of allopathy started wearing off.

Three

Encounter with a Homeopath

According to the World Health Organization (WHO) classification, homeopathy comes under Traditional and Complementary Medicine (T&CM); which is the sum total of the knowledge, skill and practices based on the theories, beliefs and experiences indigenous to different cultures, whether explicable or not, used in the maintenance of health as well as in the prevention, diagnosis, improvement or treatment of physical and mental illness, encompassing products, practices and practitioners.

As a postgraduate of Western medicine, I had a tendency to look down on traditional therapies. My initial reaction was a 'NO' to my husband's suggestion of trying homeopathy for the drug-resistant urinary tract infection that had been bugging me for some time. Traditional medicine was considered to be a psychosomatic treatment at best, and mine was not a psychiatric case. I was suffering from genuine laboratory-proven drug-resistant infection. The suggestion of trying homeopathy had come from a colleague in my husband's office who practised homeopathy as a serious hobby. He was persuasive and persistent and agreed to my demand of explaining the system to me before I tried his sugar pills.

On a hot June morning, we sat down with glasses of chilled lemonade. He was a mild and gentle soul and patiently answered all my queries. He knew that I was a newcomer who knew next to nothing about homeopathy; that I came from a world of medicine where the talk centred around blood tests and X-rays; and that I was more than a little wary about venturing into the uncharted waters of homeopathy.

Taking a sip of the lemonade, I looked at the list of questions I had made the previous day and asked him the first question, 'What is homeopathy?'

The homeopath replied, 'The name itself means "like cures like" in Greek. Homoios = similar, pathos = suffering.' He told me that this system of therapeutics focused on the patient and not on the disease or the microbe causing the disease. It is the vital stimulation of self-defence mechanisms of the living being leading to a curative, vital reaction and it aims at making the patient cure himself or herself based on the 'Law of Similars', *Similia Similibus Curanteur*.

I almost burst out laughing. To me this was unheard of. How could an infection be cured without a course of antibiotics?

Unruffled, he continued that any substance in nature, which can hurt, can also be used to cure, provided the disease has the same symptoms which that substance can cause: belladonna (a plant extract) cures scarlet fever (a bacterial infection), because the symptoms of belladonna poisoning are indistinguishable from scarlet fever. Both have the burning skin, the shining eyes with dilated pupils, the dry, sore throat, and the excitement which may lead to delirium. If snake venom causes haemorrhage then homeopathic snake venom stops haemorrhage! If poison ivy causes itching, then homeopathic poison ivy stops itching. 'Do you get it now?'

The medicine of 'Likes' sounded very interesting and intriguing to me. Seeing from my expression that I didn't get it but sensing my curiosity, he explained that the biological experiments of German Professor Hugo have also shown that where drug and disease affect tissues or cells in the same manner, identical symptoms are produced. This is known as the Similia principle and had been known since the time of Hippocrates. But it was of no practical use, as it caused aggravation in symptoms of the disease before cure took place. It became practicable only after the discovery by Dr Hahnemann (Father of Homeopathy), of preparing drugs by dilution and succussion, according to scale, in a definite proportion of drug to inert vehicle.

To my query about the scope of homeopathy, he said, 'Homeopathy is concerned with the study and administration of drugs based on the "Law of Similars". The action and scope of drugs is generated through experiments carried out on healthy human beings, and the study of toxicology and pathology. Hence, its province is only preparation and application of medicines. It presupposes a competent knowledge of anatomy, physiology, pathology, microbiology, biochemistry and diagnosis.'

My next query was how a remedy is selected in homeopathy. His reply, 'We need to figure out which remedy the patient and/or the patient's complaint resembles the most. This is done through a "homeopathic interview". The answers give the information needed—the patient's nature, likes and dislikes, and other factors, because in homeopathy, we are looking for just one thing: a remedy whose "profile" matches the patient's. We call this "constitutional prescribing", as distinct from "acute prescribing" where different information is sought. Acute medicine addresses the immediate troublesome symptom. For example, in a case of typhoid fever, a medicine selected for continuous high-grade fever may be different, it needs to be given frequently and complemented with constitutional medicine in infrequent doses.

'The drug, when prepared using the method of potentization, is called a remedy, as it has a curative action, and is capable of removing the cause of the disease. Its sources are minerals, vegetables and the animal kingdom.

'Its actions, proven on healthy human beings called "provers", are certain and known, as symptoms thus produced are meticulously recorded in a book called *Materia Medica*. These symptoms are mainly subjective, at a functional level, because the dose of the drug used is never large enough to cause a pathological change in a prover.

'Similar remedy (remedy with the same symptoms) acts at all times and under all circumstances on all living beings. It has the advantage that it can be diluted, divided and potentized at will, till the effect of treatment is gentle and rapid, and without side-effects.

'Let me give you an example. People who need the remedy *Mercurius*, which is homeopathic mercury, are very sensitive to changes in temperature, have a very narrow range of temperature-tolerance and are constantly adjusting the thermostat in the house or opening and closing windows and throwing the covers off and on in the hope of finally getting the temperature right. And what do we use mercury for in real life? Thermometers! Do you see how the patient resembles the remedy?

'This is the kind of information we hope to uncover

through the questions. If we ask you about all the things that influence you, the way you react to certain situations and people, and other things you probably think don't have anything to do with your disease, it is because we are trying to find your constitutional remedy.'

This was beginning to sound scientific and more to my liking. I asked him about the term 'Small Dose'.

Emptying his glass of lemonade, he replied, 'In employing remedies according to the principle of Similia, the quantity of dose is guided by the biological phenomena known as the "Arndt-Shultz Law". It says that "For every substance, small doses stimulate, moderate doses inhibit and large doses kill". In other words, "Weak stimuli increase physiologic activity and very strong stimuli inhibit or abolish activity".

'The infinitesimal dose in homeopathy is the result of experience and careful experiments for many years. It has its foundation in the modern scientific theory of conservation of energy and indestructibility of matter.'

'What is the homeopathic approach?' I asked. He said, 'Homeopathy, as a system, follows diagnostic criteria and approaches, as done in allopathy. Hence, the clinical history, examination techniques, findings and interpretation, investigations and criteria for prognosis are similar to allopathy. The approach to therapy, however, is distinctly different. It goes beyond clinical symptomatology into the study of the constitution of the suffering individual.

'For example, in the clinical condition of pneumonia with pleural involvement (pleurisy), chest pain, fever, cough, among other symptoms, constitute the diagnostic (common) symptoms of the disease. Some patients with pneumonia feel very thirsty especially for cold water; are excessively cold and want covering; further, the chest pain in one patient is better while lying on the same side as the pain while in another, the pain is better while lying on the painless side. These are the peculiar or characteristic symptoms a homeopathic physician is interested in, as these symptoms help him to form the totality which in turn helps in differentiating one remedy from the other.'

I looked at my watch and realized that it was almost lunchtime; thanked him for spending an entire morning. With a smile, he declined the offer of a pot-luck meal and said that the time would be well spent if I was ready to try his medicine.

Incredulous, I decided to try homeopathy, as a last resort for my problem, on the condition that he would tell me the name of the medicine that would be prescribed to me. He should also suggest the book for reading about it. After a few weeks, I had to reluctantly acknowledge the relief in pain and reduced frequency in infection. My curiosity was aroused, so, with an inclination to learn more about the subject and time on my hands, I set forth on a journey to learn a new system of therapeutics.

Four

Homeopathy Excites Interest

Life was moving at a fast pace. My husband had found a new vocation as a builder. This required full-time attention and my assistance as, for some time, he was doing dual jobs. I had a small child who also needed 24/7 looking after. In such a scenario, a full-time job or practice in medicine was not feasible. I had to be content with my part-time job, just to remain in touch with medicine. The charitable work at the Masonic Clinic would have become boring and might have led to my losing interest in it, had it not been for a newfound interest in learning about a new therapeutic system. The ups and downs of educating myself kept me mentally stimulated.

I was fond of reading, and the following years were spent in going through various books on homeopathy, besides the first three books my guide had given me: (i) James Tyler Kent's *Repertory,* which is a compilation of symptoms described in a patient's language and replicated in the number of medicines; (ii) *A Practical Dictionary of Materia Medica* by John Henry Clarke in three volumes describing all the medicines known till then; each medicine is dealt with in detail as to its source, its general mode of action, effect on each part of the body, clinical application and some case studies; (iii) *Leaders in Homeopathic Therapeutics* by E.B. Nash. This catalogues a few of the medicines that the author considers useful in daily practice. These medicines are described as a personality for easy recognition followed by their salient actions on the body. For example, the medicine *Nux vomica* is described as: *For very particular, careful, zealous persons, inclined to get excited or angry, spiteful, malicious disposition, mental workers or those having sedentary occupations. Oversensitiveness, easily offended, very little noise frightens, cannot bear the least even suitable medicine; faints easily from odours, etc...*; another medicine, *Pulsatilla*, is described as: *Mild, gentle, yielding disposition; sad and despondent, weeps easily, sandy hair, blue eyes, pale face, muscles soft and flabby.* It made an interesting read, but to find an exact replica in patients appeared a herculean task. Yet another book on *Materia Medica* called the medicine *Nux vomica predominantly a male remedy* and *Pulsatilla* as predominantly *a female remedy*. For many years, I did not understand whether this gender bias was to be strictly adhered to, or the medicines could be prescribed on their indications.

Another book on therapeutics had chapters on diseases as I knew them: abscess, anaemia, dyspepsia, sore throat, among others. Under each were described varying numbers of medicines, the indication for how and when to choose one, but it was quite vague for a beginner like me. For instance, in a case of a sore throat, it could not be ascertained as to when to use *Mercurius* or *Hepar sulphuris*. Sometimes, the patient's complaint was the hallmark (keynote symptom) of the medicine, which made the task easier. For example, the keynote symptom of *Cocculus* was car sickness, and so when someone asked to be treated for car sickness, you immediately rattled out this medicine. In moments like these, homeopathy appeared easy and magical. There was also a book available on keynote symptoms.

The sources of books were college libraries and homeopathy pharmacies; the advisors were homeopath colleagues and pharmacists. The result was that I got to read about one medicine from many *Materia Medicas* and one disease from multiple therapeutic books. Some books were favourites, and were repeatedly consulted. This continued till the digital versions came. Even now, after over forty years of medical practice, I still consult these for every patient.

There was a homeopathic pharmacy on my way to the Masonic Clinic, where I would drop by while returning from the clinic. This had become a routine, I would stop there, buy medicines, browse through the booklets placed on the table, chat with the pharmacist and pick up interesting titles.

In the initial stages of my exposure to homeopathy, I experimented with medicines as advised or learnt from books. Even then, homeopathy was mind-boggling and very confusing, to say the least. Some guidance was needed. There was a homeopathy college near my residence, which I joined sometime between 1982 and 1983, as a visiting faculty to teach modern methods of clinical diagnosis and prognosis to undergraduate students. The main idea was to come in contact with learned homeopaths and to access the college homeopathic library. The principal of the college, Dr D.P. Rastogi, sensing my interest, encouraged it and guided me. The habit of visiting pharmacies continued. After joining college, I switched to buying medicines from a pharmacy within the college premises. The pharmacist there—another chatty person, he liked to share his experiences and give tips as to which medicine was good for which disease. I enjoyed talking to him while buying medicines. The pharmacy grew and got established in the main market and remains my major supplier.

My learning was a slow process, it was not time-bound and curriculum-oriented but experience-based. I would try homeopathy in conditions where there was no specific cure in allopathy, as in skin conditions, viral infections, allergic conditions. Once, a friend asked me for medicine for itching after using hair dye. The itching was cured with couple of doses of *Sulphur*. This was interesting; I had increased my pharmacopeia of allopathy with homeopathic medicines that I had experimented with. For example, I would start treatment of coryza, a viral infection, with homeopathy but switch to antibiotics when the discharges became thick and yellowish, indicating a secondary bacterial infection, with the belief that bacterial infections could not be cured with homeopathy. While the successful cases stuck with me vividly, the failures were not registered as I would promptly switch the treatment to allopathy: as a registered postgraduate allopath.

While seeing patients at the Masonic Clinic was the only work I was doing 'officially', I soon became 'the family doctor' for relatives, friends, friends of relatives and relatives of friends, including the staff members of my husband's construction company. The feeling of being recognized as an accomplished and competent professional by friends and family was rewarding, but, as I soon discovered, it was also a double-edged sword. It seemed that there was never a 'bad time' to call. People would ring me at any and all times and launch into exhaustive and exhausting details of the colour of their urine or the mole on their hips. I was happy to provide the odd pearl of wisdom, yet, sometimes I wanted to enjoy a catch-up with friends without being asked for advice on various ailments.

Being a doctor was my calling, but becoming a homeopath was my newfound interest. I soon realized that homeopathic suggestions from an allopath were easily accepted. At the Masonic Clinic, I would give two prescriptions: one of allopathy and the other of homeopathy. I bought medicines for relatives and friends, as they had no idea how to source homeopathic medicines. Soon, I had a collection of them, which were kept in a wooden box. Gradually, the size and number of boxes increased. The wooden box was precious and travelled with me everywhere. It was particularly handy at construction sites. The staff had become used to asking for treatment for every small or big ailment and they would specifically ask for either allopathy or homeopathy. To my surprise and delight, the request for homeopathy was increasing with time.

As the number of people consulting me at home increased, it was difficult to remember their prescriptions. I got patient cards made, where patient details, date of consultation, ailment, prescription, indications for the medicine were meticulously recorded. On repeat visits, the status of the disease and efficacy of medicine was noted. This was helpful in the learning process.

Five

Learning Homeopathy

But the journey was not easy; it was fraught with many ambiguities and uncertainties. Homeopathic literature has four types of books: *Organon, Materia Medica, Therapeutics* and *Repertory. Organon* deals with the principle of homeopathy, *Similia Similibus Curanteur. Materia Medica* is the compilation of all the symptoms produced by a drug in various healthy people and from toxicology. *Therapeutics* describes the clinical conditions and various homeopathic medicines which have been found useful for that condition. *Repertory* is a compilation of symptoms as elicited in a person; the same symptom could be produced by many medicines, but in a different grade (intensity). The literature was immense; writers were many, each had his/her different way and success stories galore. It appeared that any disease could be cured by this system of therapeutics, yet, it was an enigma as to why it was shrouded in mystery and looked down upon.

After developing an interest in homeopathy, I started asking people about their awareness about it. To my surprise, there was a large number of such people. The general opinion was that it was good for skin diseases and 'if it worked', could give miraculous results, when every other treatment failed. The literature was full of such stories, but there were no protocols for practitioners to achieve results on a regular basis. For the same disease different experts could advise different medicines. Also, the same medicine could be good for a simple headache, sunstroke, meningitis or scarlet fever. I realized that in spite of the vast literature, there was no easy protocol for making a prompt prescription and guidelines for the management of a disease. The physician was left on his/her own to find out the nature of the disease and the perfect medicine.

The main tool for diagnosis and treatment in homeopathy was the history of the disease, which is essentially the same as in allopathy. Allopathy relied on various types of investigation for treatment; in homeopathy it was the correct assessment of the symptoms, their modalities and characteristic combination that diagnose the correct similimum for the treatment. In the beginning I didn't understand the logic of asking many questions, for example, the logic of asking about the desire for sweets or savouries in a case of asthma; desire for hot/cold drinks in eczema and if cold drinks, whether chilled or at room temperature; sleeping position: sleeping on the right side or left or back or tummy, with arms over the head or under the head, with arms and legs wide apart or in knee-chest position; site/ degree of perspiration and importance of mental symptoms. For selection of certain medicines, even the history of sexual behaviour was important. It was overwhelming and embarrassing to the patient as well as for me.

Once, a middle-aged gentleman came for consultation for a complicated problem. He was distantly related, though a complete stranger to me, the relationship being akin to that with a son-in-law (if you are an Indian, you will appreciate the delicateness). The interrogation started with great enthusiasm for finding the correct remedy, then got stuck in the choice between two medicines, which could only be solved by asking about sexual behaviour (at that time). I was so psyched that I blurted out the question. He was a polished man, holding a high position. With a cool demeanour he answered, but I was embarrassed. Even today I turn pink, thinking about the incident.

A nine-year-old boy was brought for complaints of retrosternal (centre of the chest) pain, offensive burping, tummy ache and frequent stools, triggered by eating chicken and dairy products. These were the only foods he desired and couldn't be stopped from eating them. Now, for finding the right medicine, I had to ask questions about burping, bloating as well as the type, colour and smell of his stool. The boy resented this and said to his mother, 'Mom, I don't want to visit that doctor. She asks such awkward questions.'

A young couple came for consultation. The man said that his wife was sick, they were tired of frequent use of antibiotics and wanted to try homeopathy. I asked the lady, 'What's your problem?' She said, 'You tell me what my problem is?' The man helpfully intervened to say that she suffered from frequent pain in the throat. During such episodes, she stopped eating and was very irritable. This was not sufficient information for me to find the right medicine. What to do? It appeared that homeopathy is not meant for everyone. However, training in modern medicine helped me. Clinical examination of the patient revealed that the condition of the throat matched with the description of the same in a particular homeopathic medicine, and the patient got over her problem without the use of antibiotics.

An elderly lady came for the treatment of long-standing eczema of the foot. For many years it was effectively controlled with the use of local ointments in modern medicine. Homeopathic treatment required some detailed questioning. Her husband had recently retired from a very senior position in the Indian Railways, hence she was used to being pampered rather than questioned. Homeopathic questioning overwhelmed her and she kept saying, 'Why are you asking these questions? I am normal, there is nothing wrong with me and this is just a superficial skin problem.'

I had read in *Organon* that if the symptoms of the patient matched with the symptoms of the medicine, as given in *Materia Medica,* one dose of the medicine would remove all the symptoms and cure the disease. A twenty-year-old lady came to me one Saturday complaining about a recurrent sore throat for the last few years. The sore throat was effectively treated with allopathic medicine, but she was tired of taking antibiotics. I thought that she was a good candidate on whom to try homeopathy. With her consent, I noted all her symptoms and found that *Hep. 30c* matched her condition perfectly and advised her to take one dose of the medicine. Ten days later, she reported that by the same evening, her condition had worsened, with fever and a painful swelling in the throat, compelling her to take her usual allopathic medicine. Going back to homeopathic literature, I found that a lower potency (dilution) helped in ripening of infection and a higher potency aborted it. Next time, along with *200c,* a second prescription of allopathy was also given, in the eventuality of the previous episode recurring. This was the beginning of my giving two prescriptions to my patients: one allopathic, the other homeopathic. I was perplexed as the same sequence of events was repeated. Going back to the literature, I found that another medicine, *Merc-i-r.*, matched the symptoms, which had developed after taking *Hep.* Third time two prescriptions were given: first, homeopathy with two medicines, *Merc-i-r.*, to be taken twice a day, afternoon and evening, and *Hep.* in the next morning. The second, allopathy, was a bystander. The feedback from the patient was positive; she had not needed a second prescription.

Repetition/changing the medicine was of great importance in the art and science of homeopathy.

A patient with an eczematous lesion near his left knee joint came for treatment. Based on the symptoms, I prescribed *Sulph. 30c,* one dose a day for three days, along with an allopathic skin ointment. By the next week the lesion had healed completely. Three months later, he came back again with the same lesion at the same spot but slightly bigger in size, and informed me that the use of the earlier medicine and ointment had not been helpful, though the symptoms were exactly same. As per the directions of *Organon,* I was required to give a dose of higher potency, which was *Sulph. 200c.* It was a dilemma for two reasons: one was a reference by homeopathy writer E.B. Nash who had vividly described aggravation with *Sulph. 200c,* the second was a horror story of homeopathic aggravation, told by my sister-in-law who was a paediatrician at Post Graduate Institute (PGI), Chandigarh, and her strong condemnation of homeopathy. My faith in Hahnemann's logic overpowered the confusion and I prescribed *Sulph. 200c* with explicit instructions to take ONE DOSE ONLY and consult me after two days so that I could monitor any aggravation. The patient did not come for ten days and each day was a nightmare for me. I imagined and dreamt that the patient had gone to Chandigarh, he had developed aggravation, landed at PGI Hospital and everyone was asking him the name of the fool who had prescribed homeopathy. On the tenth day, the patient walked into the clinic. He looked well, sat down and showed me his left knee. There was no sign of any lesion. He confirmed that he had taken one dose and asked for further instructions. I was confused and wanted him to explain. He said that he had been taking only one dose a day for the last ten days and enquired for how long was he required to continue this wonderful medicine.

My fear of *Sulph. 200c* potency and repetition evaporated. I have been prescribing *Sulphur* frequently and fearlessly, but strictly on its indications.

The general impression about homeopathic treatment was that it was very restrictive. People who believed in this therapy, and wanted to follow it, felt that there were too many dos and don'ts attached to the treatment. This hampered the routine and was inconvenient to follow. Initially, I would add homeopathy to mainstream treatment, only when convinced of its usefulness, without imposing any restrictions. I thought that a medicine had to be more potent than the diet; but a doubt lurked in my mind as to its efficacy on two accounts: (i) on the minuteness of dose and (ii) on not observing the rules mentioned in the *Organon*. One day, I came across a booklet: 'Dietetic restrictions in homeopathic practice', written by a famous homeopath, Dr P. Sankaran, which put to rest all the doubts. He had very convincingly laid to rest the futility of dietary restrictions, citing his experiences and those of many other successful homeopaths.

Gradually I developed a system of arriving at the seemingly right medicine. I first read about the disease in one of the therapeutic books, Kent's *Repertory*, then went through all the medicines listed therein in a *Materia Medica* book and choose the medicine that matched the most. It was arduous and time-consuming but could be rewarding. One of my relatives had suffered from nasal polyps for many years. He had been operated upon a few years ago, but the polyps had recurred, causing nasal obstruction, breathing difficulty and insomnia for the last two years. Poor man! He could not lie down for more than two hours at a stretch. He had to take steam inhalations before lying down again and sleeping. Surgical excision was not feasible, as the polyps were too many and too widely spread. In Kent's *Repertory*, five medicines were listed. I read about all five in Clarke's *Materia Medica*, and chose one that appeared to be the most suited. After two days of four pills three times a day, he slept non-stop for twenty-four hours. His next complaint was that if he slept like this, then when would he work? His words were an elixir to my ears and all the long hours spent on one patient were forgotten. His treatment took two years before the nasal obstruction was completely cured with changes in medicines according to symptoms.

I was amazed at the potential of homeopathy. Of course, it was arduous and time-consuming, but I had all the time and inclination. Though, such a result was few and far between, it typically happened when I was about to give up homeopathy as a bad choice. The thought, 'Why did I have to get into an ambiguous system of medicine when I have the license to practise a system of accepted efficacy?' was effectively countered by the occurrence of such cases and they renewed my resolve to study the system in-depth and be convinced of its efficacy.

Six

Ups and Downs In Practice

I had resolved to study the system in-depth to convince myself of its efficacy. In the initial stages of my exposure to homeopathy, I experimented with medicines as advised or learned from books. But, I was an allopath, hence, I viewed the results of therapy from the eye of an allopath. The results of homeopathic medicine had to be as fast and perceptible, as with modern medicine; otherwise, I would switch to allopathy. Though the increase in my pharmacopeia of homeopathic medicines gave me an added advantage and a high, yet allopathy remained the mainstay of my practice. Whenever there was a patient, who either showed an unsatisfactory response to treatment or needed too many medicines for multiple symptoms, I tried adding homeopathic medicines with the patient's approval. The result was two prescriptions: one of allopathy for the diagnosed disease and the other of homeopathy for symptomatic relief. Though there were two prescriptions, yet the total number of medicines was less and compliance was more. My popularity increased and I became known as the 'two prescriptions doctor'.

Each case treated with homeopathy alone or in

combination with allopathy was a learning process for me. I observed the result and made comparisons with what had been achieved with only allopathy. Some cases left a permanent impression. These are detailed below, with the learning and observation from them.

Homeopathy can be complementary to allopathy

My learning of homeopathy began with *Leaders In Homeopathic Therapeutics* by E.B. Nash. It opened with a description of *Nux vomica*. I found it an unusual, but interesting, way to describe a medicine. That same week a patient came to the clinic with complaints of dyspepsia, irritability and restless sleep, and a BP (blood pressure) reading of 140/100 mm. I was about to write the prescription, when the patient informed that he did not want any sedative as it led to unrefreshing sleep, and an antihypertensive drug made him so weak that he could not attend to his work. I prescribed *Nux-v. 30c*, one dose in the evening for seven days. Next week, all his symptoms were absent, except for acidity, BP was 125/85 mm. Surprised, I prescribed *Nux-v. 30c*, two doses a day for seven days. A week later he came back happy as there were no symptoms, except for slight heaviness of the head and a BP reading of 135/95. Both doctor and patient were pleased with the outcome and the patient agreed to take a small dose of an antihypertensive medication. For the next few years his treatment with both systems continued successfully.

Observation: The impression that homeopathy and allopathy could not be used at the same time was shaken. Homeopathy could give symptomatic relief but for treatment of hypertension conventional medicine was required. After that, I managed many cases of diabetes and hypertension with two prescriptions, one of allopathy and the second of homeopathy, with increased patient compliance and satisfaction.

'Three doses doctor'

- A middle-aged man from the nearby market came to me with a complaint of eruptions on the scalp. I prescribed three doses of a homeopathic medicine (don't remember the name) and within a short time the scalp was clear. Thereafter, I came to be known as the 'three doses doctor'.

- A forty-five-year-old man came to me with complaints of periodic headaches of many years' duration which had been diagnosed as a case of migraine. The episodes would occur every three to four weeks. The results of all his investigations had come within normal limits. He had suffered from pulmonary tuberculosis (TB) before the start of the present condition, which was fully treated with conventional antitubercular antibiotics. I gave him three doses of a homeopathic medicine, matching with his complaints and past history, and next month and thereafter, his headaches did not return.

Observation: Impressive result, unexplainable with my current knowledge.

- A distressed father of an eight-month-old male infant, once asked for medicine for the child. The complaint was of frequent stools since the last two months. The child was in the dentition phase and in the habit putting everything into his mouth. Many paediatricians (child specialists) had been consulted, resulting in short-term improvement each time. But now the child had lost his appetite because of frequent medicines which had not controlled the frequency of stools. I had recently read about a medicine called *Podophyllum* which could be used to treat frequent light-coloured offensive smelling stools—same as the child—and was effective in dentition diarrhoea. One dose of two small pills controlled the frequency promptly, but he was given two more doses at a twelve hours' interval, with instructions to give a dose at the beginning of the diarrhoea. Thereafter, the dentition phase went smoothly.

Observation: Homeopathy is effective and safe for children.

- A thirty-four-year-old lady had had a caesarean on 24 July 1996. On 17 August, she developed fever, which rose sharply to 104° F within three hours. The fever was preceded by chills, a severe headache, and her entire body felt sore and bruised. There was excruciating pain in the whole body on nursing her child. Two days prior to the onset of fever, the weather had become cold and very damp due to continuous rains. She had washed a lot of clothes and had caught a chill. The patient's left breast was swollen, red-hot, hard and very tender; her left arm movement was painful; but there was no stitch abscess.

The disease picture matched closely with the drug picture of a homeopathic medicine, *Phytolacca*. With the patient's consent, I prescribed it against the practice of giving antibiotics. To my surprise, and everyone's delight, the fever and swelling reduced with one dose. However, the patient took two more doses in the fear of the fever coming back again. I asked her to stop the medicine.

Observation: Homeopathy is fast-acting and can be as effective as antibiotics.

- A thirty-six-year-old lady had had a normal first delivery three weeks ago. The episiotomy incision (surgical cut to facilitate delivery) given at the time of birthing had apparently healed well, but the patient continued to have severe pain around the area. Three courses of antibiotics were not helpful. The pain was quite intolerable, particularly when sitting. I visited the patient in the evening; she was lying down, tight-lipped with a frown on her face. There was no fever or any other complaint. On examination, I found the wound had healed well, but the skin around the scar was stretched, glazed and very tender, without any swelling, fluctuation or pus point. She asked for dinner, and when it came, she was helped to sit up. Suddenly she winced and pushed the tray away and was rude and snappish. The food had been of the patient's choice, cooked by her mother. The scene reminded me of a homeopathy medicine. Next morning, one dose of *Staph. 30c* was given at eleven o'clock. It made the patient feverish and chilly; it was repeated after four hours at three o'clock, following which the patient had fever with chills. The medicine was stopped and hydrotherapy started. The fever continued to rise and a swelling developed at the labial end of the scar, which burst open in the early hours of the next day and a bowlful of foul pus was discharged. In the morning, the patient had a smile on her face, in spite of a gruelling night, and was thankful for the treatment.

Observation: The effect of a few small, sweet pills was almost magical. I was impressed with the result of the *Similia* principle and resolved to pursue the study of homeopathy more seriously. To that end, I became an associate member of the Faculty of Homeopathy, London, in 1991.

Long-term management of marasmus

- A friend of mine was very worried. Her only grandchild had fainted again in school. The frequency of her fainting spells was increasing. She was a pretty six-year-old girl of delicate constitution, who had recently joined regular school. During the assembly, the children had to stand in the open; the heat and the crowds would make her faint and she would be sent back home. These episodes were followed by fever and convulsions, which were scary. She was the only child of an affluent family who had been overmedicated with the conventional treatment; in addition, all types of prayers in various temples had been carried out. My friend said that she had faith in homeopathy, but her daughter was against it. Together, we planned a strategy to combine the two systems of therapeutics: homeopathy to be used on a regular basis and allopathic treatment for fever, diarrhoea and vomiting.

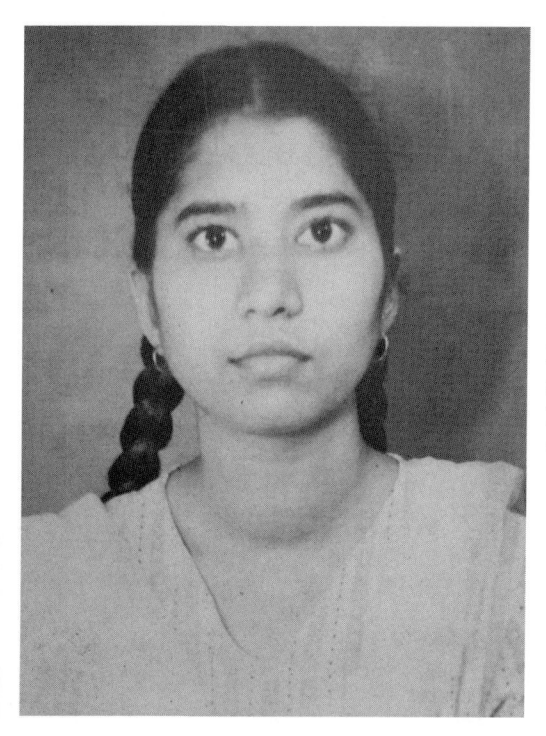

The author as a young biology student (*top left*): an initial dislike for dissection turned into a passion for anatomy studies in medical school; and (*below*) with her grandfather, who said, 'Let the girl become a doctor'.

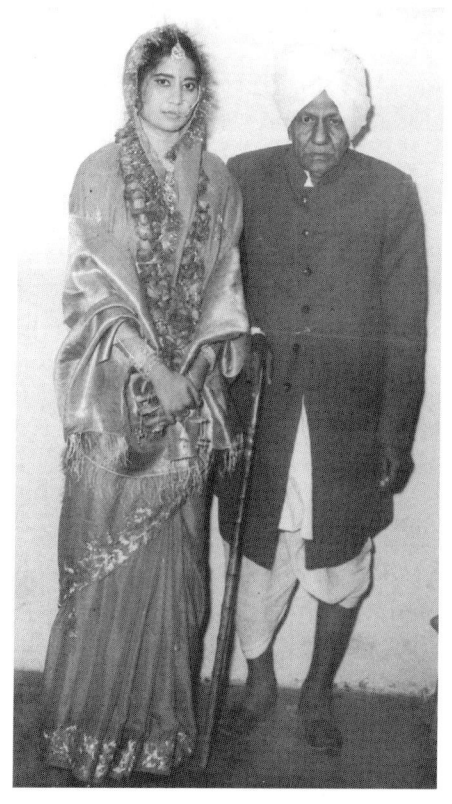

All images courtesy Kusum Chand

GOLDEN JUBILEE (1964 - 2014)

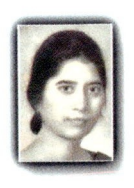

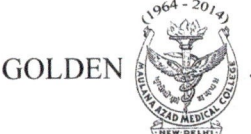

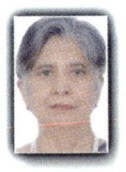

Dr Kusum Jain

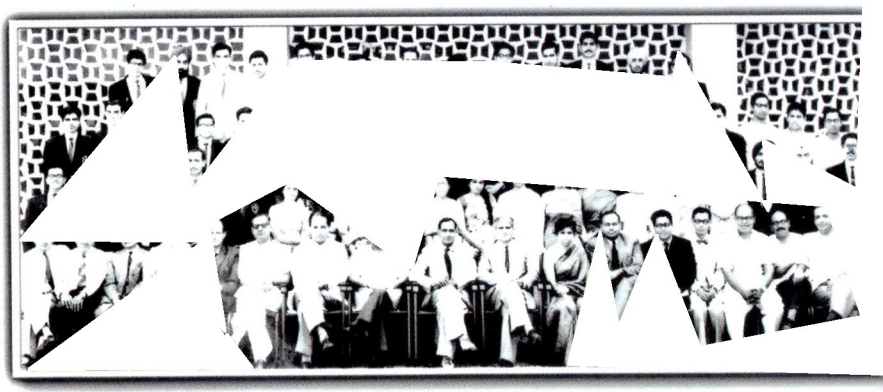

Left to Right Sitting :- Dr Vishnu Kumar , Dr Ved Prakash , Dr M L Sharma , Dr R K Sanyal , Dr DN Gupta , Dr Ramesh Nigam , Dr H Vaishnav , Dr BP Sinha , Col BL Taneja
  Maj Gen BN Bhandari , Dr A Dass , Dr SP Jain , Dr SRK Malik , Dr R Sen , Dr A K Banerjee , Dr H K Chuttani , Dr K C Mahajan

Standing 1st Row :- N Kasturirangan , D P Manandhar, A K Karnik , S L Vohra, Dev Prakash, Renu Kapoor, Saroj Gandhi, Indu Mago, Lata Vad, Shameem Akhtar, Veena Gupta
  Asha Singh , Bina Seghal , Radha S Motwani , Santosh K Chojar , Kusum Jain , Cuckoo Bhatnagar , Santosh Kapoor , Jagjit Singh , J B Singh , R K Kapila

Standing 2nd Row :- S N A Rizvi , R K Bhatia, S K Gupta, J C Dang, R S Misra, Surender Mohan, Balak Ram, N R Joshi, R K Arora , H V Kumar, Raghubir Singh
  Nirmal Chander, O P Chitkara, Mohd. Afzal, M Y S Ballawy, G N Bhatt, P C Chamyal, Vinod S Saxena, S P Gupta , Y P Gupta

Standing 3rd Row :- Raj K Gupta , Harmit Singh , H R Yadav , P L Puri, Y C Mahajan , V R Anand , R K Gupta , Y P Munjal , S C Gulati , S D Khanna , H Grover , H S Nagi , G L Arora

The author with her Class of 1964; the photograph was presented to her 50 years later at the Golden Jubilee Celebrations. Kusum Chand is fourth from right in the first row (*standing*)

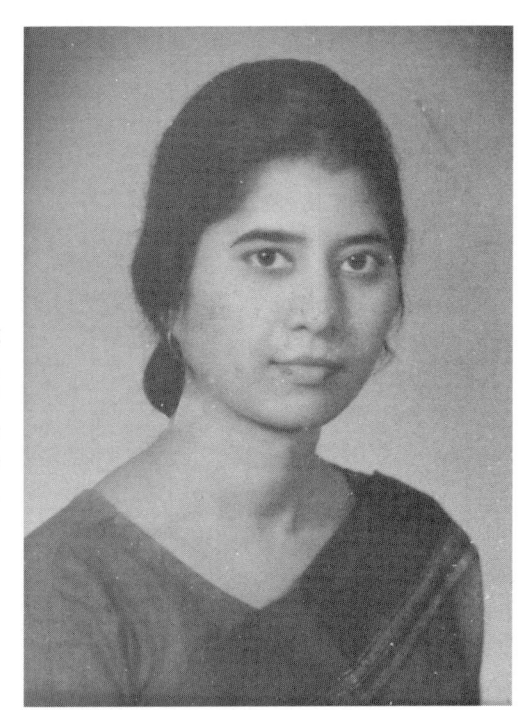

Kusum Chand as a young medico (*top right*) and, (*below*) the 'suitable boy' who was not averse to letting his wife practise medicine.

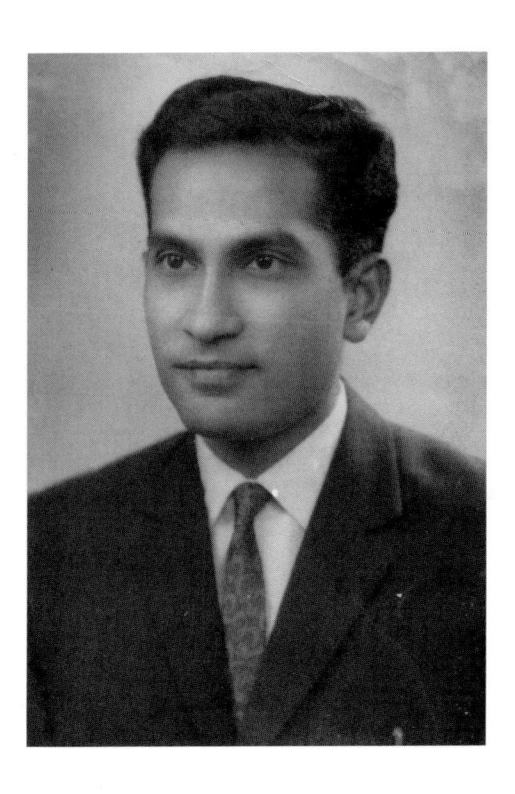

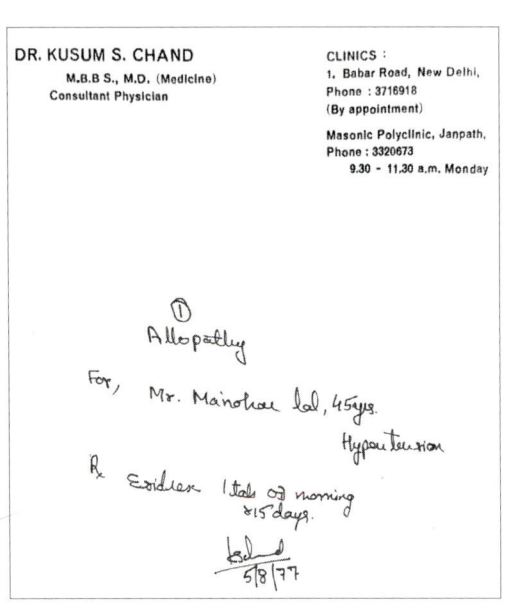

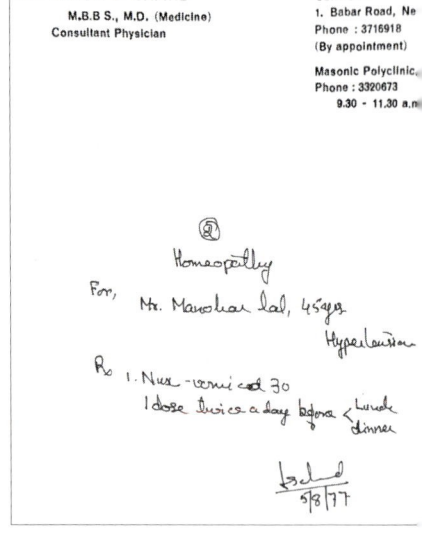

The 'two-prescription doctor'—Kusum Chand at the Masonic Polyclinic, Janpath, New Delhi

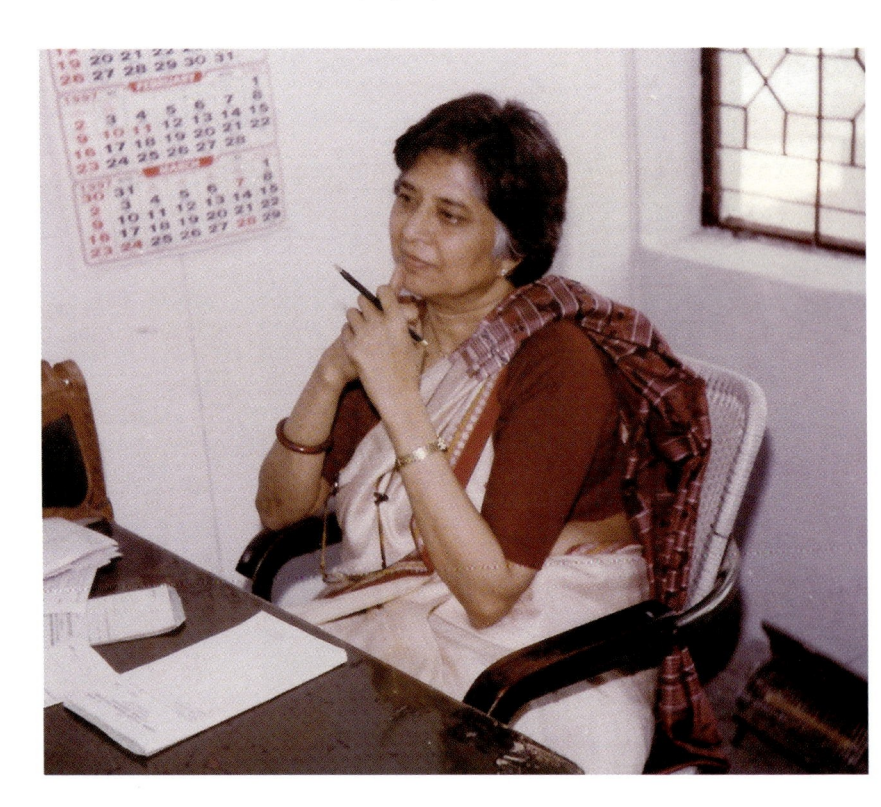

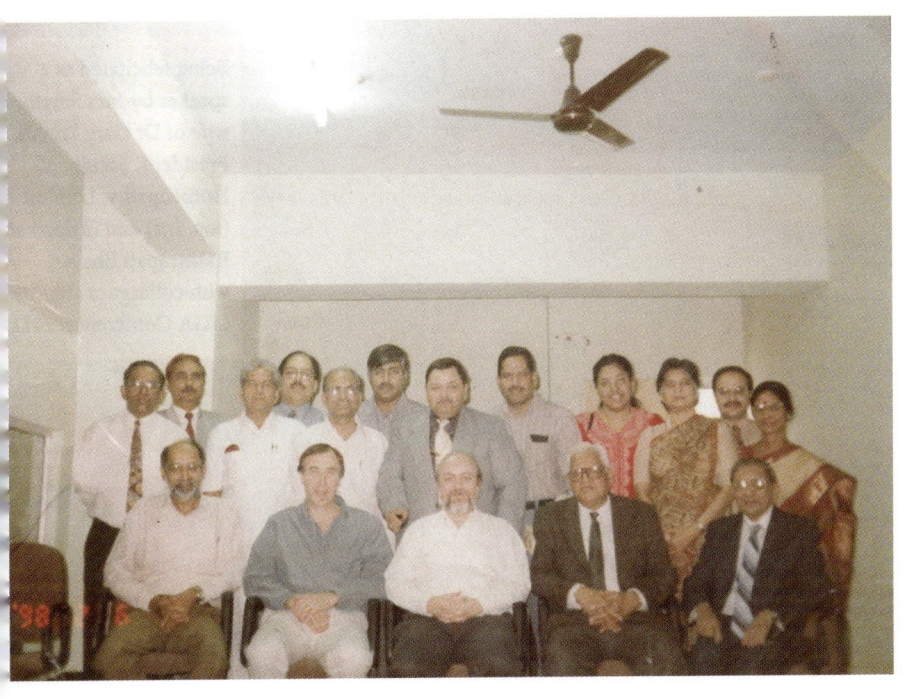

Finally, a homeopath!
With the batch of 1998. Kusum Chand is standing in the last row, second from right.

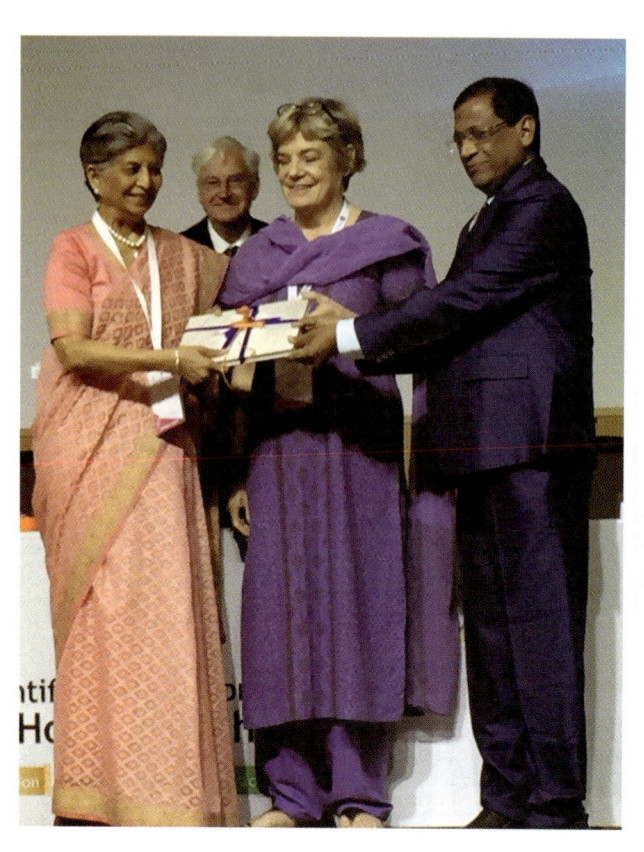

Being felicitated as a speaker by Dr. Helen Beaumont - Medical Dean, The Faculty of Homeopathy in 2019 *(Top Left)* and at Rashtrapati Bhavan with colleagues after the LIGA Conference in 2011 *(Below)*

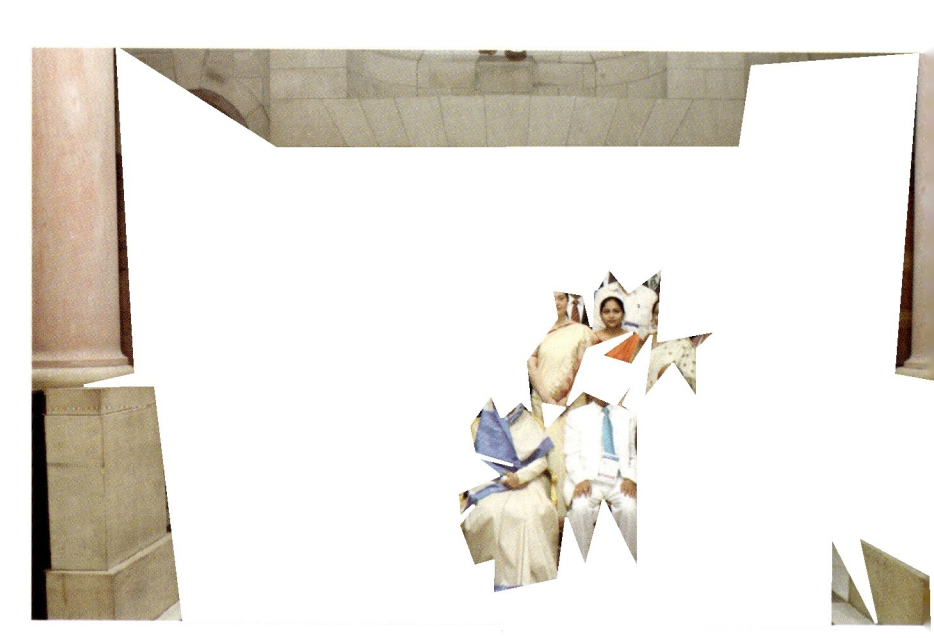

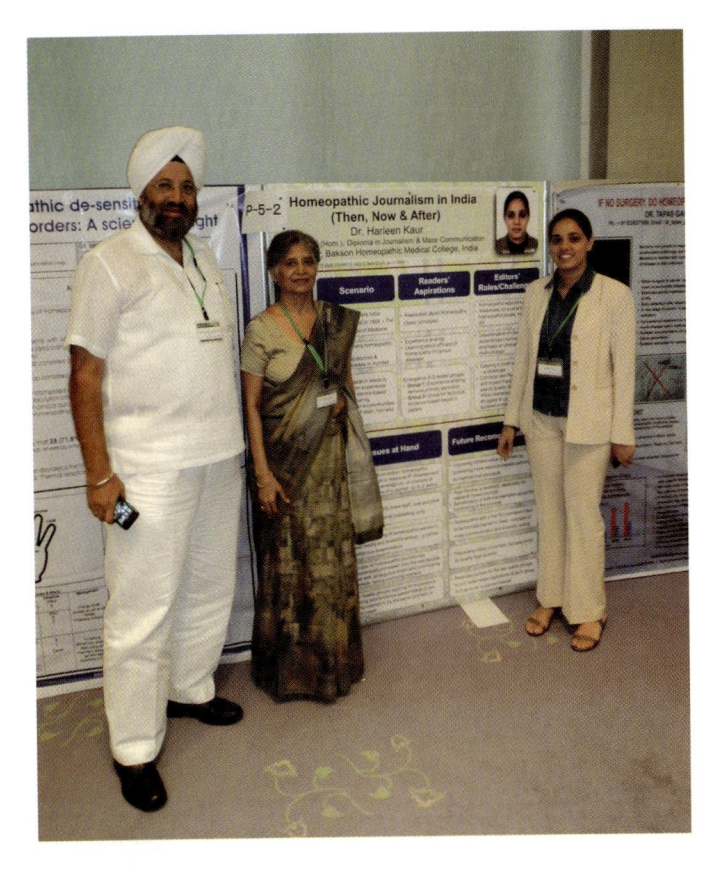

At the LIGA Conference, Japan, 2012, with Dr S.P.S. Bakshi and Dr H. Kaur, (*above*) and (*below*) at Max Vaishali with Dr Priya Kapoor

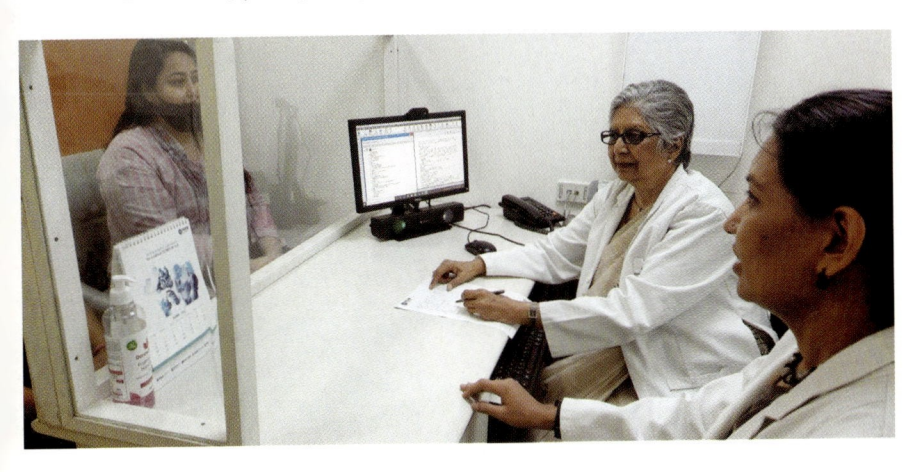

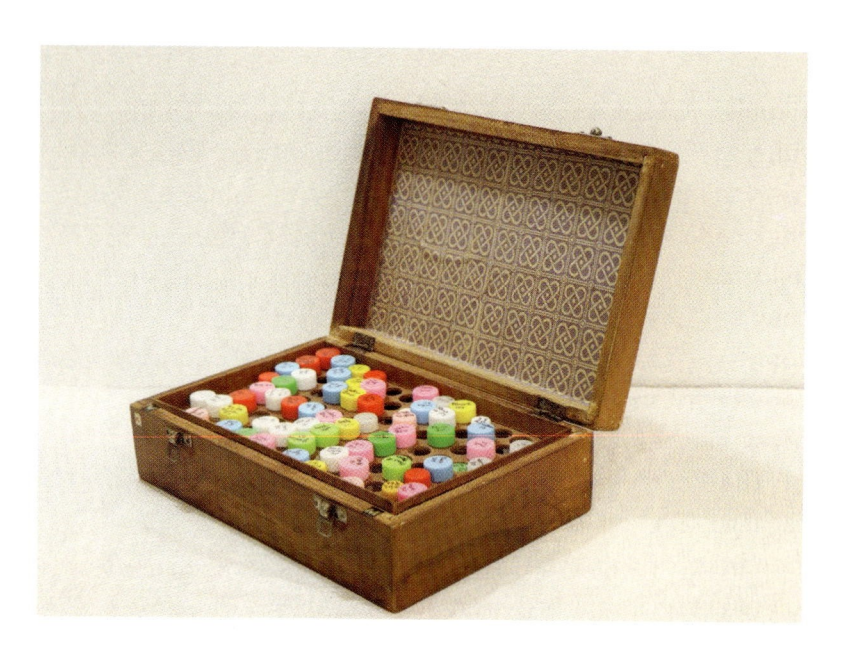

The author's famous 'travelling pillbox' (*above*), and (*below*) at her home clinic

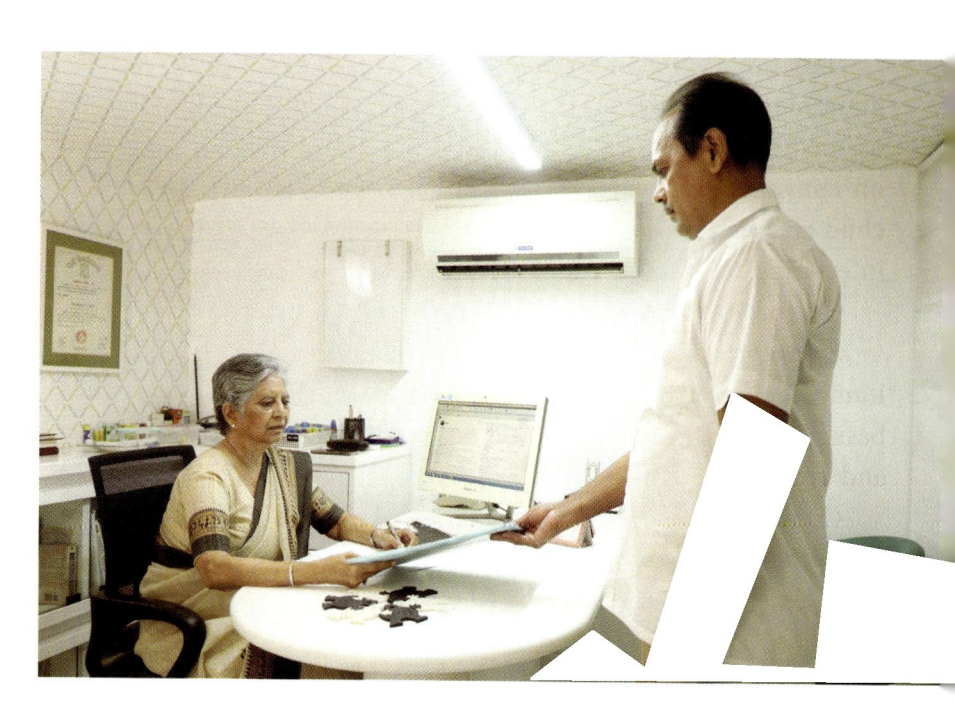

I took a detailed history and found that the child also suffered from frequent episodes of diarrhoea which was triggered by even the slightest exposure to cold, rich food, anger and dentition. She frequently had a running nose, followed by pain in the throat and a suffocating paroxysmal cough, with rattling mucous, the paroxysm often ending in vomiting. Travelling made her sick and she would often vomit. The child was emaciated, with stunted growth and frizzy hair, though the milestones were normal.

The child was carrying a lot of genetic and familial baggage. There was a family history of TB in her maternal grandmother, who was allergic to cats; her mother too was full of allergies and had been hospitalized for the most part of her pregnancy. Her father had *Streptococcus haemolyticus* (a bacterial infection), sore throat and frequent episodes of sinusitis.

Treatment was carried out with the help of her grandmother, my friend. In the beginning both systems of medicine were operative. The child's mother insisted on conventional medicine, but she soon realized that her child was benefiting more from homeopathy and stopped interfering.

The patient was managed at three levels:

Symptomatic treatment was used in frequent doses for immediate relief of symptoms on an as-and-when-required basis: *Bell. 30c* for headache and fever; *Ip. 30c* for diarrhoea and cough.

Constitutional treatment was based on the reaction of the patient to her environment; it was used at regular intervals (weekly, fortnightly) even when the patient was well: *Calc-p. 30c* in single doses.

Tubercular dyscrasia (family history of TB and allergy):

Bac. 200c, three doses at monthly intervals followed by *Tub. 1M* at three-monthly intervals.

With regular use of constitutional medicine, the symptomatic medicines were more effective. After the dose of *Bac.*, the frequency and severity of the diarrhoea and cough/cold reduced markedly. Her appetite returned, and the patient started assimilating food. In a year's time, she had gained weight, and height and her hair too had become shiny and luxuriant.

Observation: Homeopathy could not only treat symptoms of disease but could also be curative in inherited dyscrasia.

Treatment of lifestyle disorders—obesity

- A forty-five-year-old man came to me with the complaint that he had been diagnosed recently with hypertension and was put on conventional medication, which he was averse to taking on a long-term basis and wanted an alternate option. He was obese, addicted to tobacco and had many excuses for not going for regular morning walks. I prescribed, on the basis of physical and mental generals, his constitutional homeopathic medicine, *Sulph. 30c,* one dose once a day, and advised him to continue with the conventional medicine as before. Within three months he had become regular with his morning walks, so much so that he would go for a walk even in rain, his weight had reduced and tobacco chewing was substantially less. He stopped all medication and continued with lifestyle changes, with regular though infrequent use of homeopathy.

For the last twelve years, he has maintained his blood pressure with improved eating habits, yoga and morning walks.

Observation: Early intervention with homeopathy helps in making and adhering to lifestyle changes. This delays onset of irreversible chronic diseases.

Along with symptoms, biochemical constants are also corrected

- A twenty-five-year-old man came with acute pain on the left side of the face, radiating to the ears, head and teeth; associated with mild fever and unsteadiness of gait. He had been suffering for a month from cold and cough, accompanied by profuse thick, creamy, and occasionally bloody, discharge from the throat and nose in the morning. Treatment with antibiotics, analgesics and anti-allergic medicines had been effective and the expectoration had become scanty, when he developed this pain. Addition of homeopathic medicines used earlier did not help.

Examination revealed: Temperature 100° F; haemoglobin 14.4 g/dl; total leukocytic count 6,700/dl, neutrophils 41%, lymphocytes 31%, eosinophils 21% (absolute count 1407), monocytes 07%; and bilateral maxillary sinusitis on radiology. *Verb. 30c,* one dose three times a day, was selected for left-sided trigeminal neuralgia with maxillary sinusitis.

There was a remarkable improvement with the first dose itself. I repeated the medicine twice more. One week later, the leukocyte counts were repeated for curiosity's sake, as the patient was much improved. Total leukocyte count 5900/dl, neutrophils 38%, lymphocytes 35%, eosinophils 06% (absolute count 354), monocytes 01%. The patient was advised to take a dose of *Verb. 30c* on recurrence of pain.

- My pathologist friend contacted me for an oozing lesion on her left great toe; the discharge was a sticky yellowish fluid. She had taken two rounds of antibiotics on the advice of a dermatologist without any lasting effect. Cortisone cream caused an intense burning sensation. Oral steroids were prescribed which she was reluctant to take. I prescribed *Graph. 30c* three times a day for three days. On the third day, a thick scab had formed and the oozing was much less. She was advised to continue the treatment for a week. To our pleasant surprise, the lesion had healed completely, leaving a normal soft skin. After two months, she noticed that her bouts of sneezing in the morning had reduced substantially. When she checked her blood for eosinophil count, it had reduced from usual 15% to 5%

Observation: Homeopathy is fast-acting and corrects biochemical abnormality along with symptoms.

Such cases, though few and far between, convinced me of the usefulness of this therapeutic system to the extent that I took pride in calling myself a homeopath, forgetting the general impression in the public psyche that homeopathy is good for only hair fall, warts and dark/white spots on the skin. Hence, I was frequently confronted with these questions; this was vexing, particularly in social gatherings. Typically, a gentleman would start a conversation by asking about my vocation in life. My reply would be that I was a doctor. 'What specialty?' 'I am a physician, but practise homeopathy.' Condescendingly, with a long sympathetic look he would say, 'Oh, how nice! You are the right person to help me out with this little problem of hair fall.' 'Do you have any other problem?' 'I am a healthy person; just have seasonal attacks of cold and sore throat, which are effectively controlled with a small pill and nasal spray/inhaler (with steroid).' This would leave me with a dilemma. In modern medicine, there is a specialist for each part of the body, while homeopathy is a holistic medicine. For treating hair fall, I would have to consider the respiratory allergy, which the patient did not understand. Also, hair fall could be the effect of the medicines. Even if the gentleman is aware of it, he expects you to prevent hair fall without stopping the allergy treatment. Similarly, a lady after giving me that sympathetic quizzical look would ask about a brown spot on her face. 'Do you have anything in homeopathy for this little spot?' even though her disease was being handled efficiently (according to the lady) by a very experienced gynaecologist.

Acknowledging the efficacy of homeopathy was another block in the public psyche. When confronted with a case declared incurable by the dominant system of therapeutics—allopathy—people, at least in India, have a tendency to look towards alternate systems of therapeutics. But they were still reluctant to accept the good effect.

I was summoned by an elderly friend. Her son-in-law was suffering from an anal fissure, a very painful condition. He was advised surgery, which he was reluctant to undergo.

His physician suggested homeopathy as an alternative, hence the summons. I took up the challenge and with great zeal selected the medicine and mode of giving it. This was prepared in liquid form and a bottle was given. Two days later, another bottle was requested, which was complied with, without any update on pain. The third time I ventured to ask about the status of the pain. The wife promptly replied, 'Oh! I have been giving him papaya regularly and he has no pain now.' Now, if papaya was the medicine, why was a homeopath summoned?

- A friend called me on a Sunday evening and said that his mother was suffering from a terminal liver disease. The doctors at the hospital had given up, she had been brought home and could I do something. Next day, I went to see the patient, an obese lady. She was in a stupor, but responding to stimuli; there was a big burn mark on her abdomen from frequent hot applications. A liquid preparation comprising few suitable medicines was made. To my surprise, she responded well and within two weeks was playing cards with friends. This fact was not shared with me, only the request for medicine had stopped. At a later date, when I met them and enquired about the health of their mother, I was informed that Mansarover Lake water was the reason for recovery.

Observation: Now, when they had this magic water then why call for a homeopath?

These patient interactions both enriched my understanding of an alternative system of medicine, as also the complexities of therapeutic response, though some interactions did leave me vexed at the patronizing and toffee-nosed attitude towards homeopathy. But, since I had by now gauged that contending with sceptics and critics is something of a time-honoured tradition for a homeopath, my faith and interest remained strong. The ups and downs in experimenting and learning went on for more than two decades.

Seven

Dilemma: To Be or Not To Be

More than two decades of walking the path of being a physician, a homeopath and, an allopath-cum-homeopath, had left me richer in terms of both clinical experience and positive experiences in homeopathy. The most wonderful moments were when I would hear from a patient, 'I am much, much better now.' The numerous hours of reading, of homeopathic repertorization (the technique of finding a suitable medicine by using a *Repertory*, see p. 20) and of researching would become worth the effort! The persistent popularity of homeopathy, against the odds of the factory-like system of conventional allopathic medicine, steadily led to the 'little white pills', making more sense to me.

The results of being a 'two prescriptions' doctor were satisfying. The number of homeopathic prescriptions kept increasing, till a time came when they outnumbered prescriptions of allopathic medicine. I was getting convinced of the efficacy of homeopathy, particularly in a general practice. The switch over to homeopathy from allopathy was a big step. There were times when I was in a dilemma, more so, when stray events hurt the ego. As a postgraduate in medicine, one was looked up to. However, when I prescribed only homeopathy and insisted on it (convinced that it was better for the patient), I was told that a doctor (proper doctor) had also been consulted, implying that a homeopath was not a doctor.

That set me thinking: who is a doctor? A qualified practitioner, who is adept in the art and science of restoration and preservation of health, he/she does so by applying the knowledge that was learned as a student and subsequently gathered from experience. A patient seeks the advice of such a doctor when he/she is not able to endure the discomfort caused by a disease and is unable to carry out the normal routine of life. A sense of fear/insecurity, as to the safety of life, creeps into the psyche of the person. A good doctor analyses the cause of the disease and suggests corrective measures, which may range from nutrients, exercise, immunity boosters, drugs and change in lifestyle.

Knowledge and preparation of drugs is the science of pharmacology. Medicinal substances have been gathered from many sources, ranging from plants, minerals, insects and animals. The method of preparation and application of medicinal substances differs in different parts of the world, at different times over the millennia, leading to the evolution of many therapeutic systems. While each system is useful, it is not ubiquitous and does not completely satisfy all the needs of a patient in the various stages of a disease, or the vast array of diseases encountered by a human being during his lifetime.

I had become fairly conversant with two therapeutic systems—allopathy and homeopathy—and at that point in time, was confused over the choice. While teaching final year students of a homeopathic medical college, a comparison of treatment protocol of the two systems struck me.

Which system of medicine?

As far as the patient is concerned, he/she wants to be free of the sickness in the easiest and quickest possible way, no matter what the system is. The first preference may be influenced by the previous conditioning of the mind. But if one system does not offer the desired relief, the patient is quick to change the doctor or the system.

Here is an example of a case of sore throat. This is a common disease; the incidence rate is 25.7%.

A seven-year-old male child is brought with complaints of fever, acute pain in the throat and inability to eat due to pain on swallowing. He had slept the previous night in a reasonable state of health, except that he had been lethargic the whole day from playing in the sun and did not have a proper dinner. He had moderate fever and a flushed face. He is the only child of two educated working parents, who are worried and anxious as the child had been getting these attacks too frequently.

Allopathic system of medicine

After taking the history, a clinical examination is carried out and the following points are noted:

Temperature—103°F, pulse—124/mt. regular

Throat—red, congested and swollen tonsils

Clinical diagnosis—acute tonsillitis

Investigations—Blood for Total Leukocyte Count (TLC) and Differential Leukocyte Count (DLC); throat swab for microscopic examination and culture/sensitivity test

Prescription:

1. Anti-inflammatory drug (to bring down temperature (temp.), so that the patient is comfortable and to prevent febrile convulsions
2. Anti-allergic drug
3. Cold sponging (to keep temp. below 102° F)
4. Temp. and pulse chart
5. Plenty of fluids
6. Review after investigations

Twenty-four hours later:

TLC and DLC show changes of acute inflammation

Throat swab shows preponderance of one particular type of microbe.

Prescription: Empirically selected antibiotic is added on the presumption that bacteria would be sensitive to it.

Forty-eight hours later, after the culture and drug sensitivity report, either the same antibiotic is continued or changed. Doctor is concerned with the diagnosis of acute bacterial tonsillitis, emphasizes the seriousness of the disease to the worried and anxious parents. Advises them to diligently follow the full course of antibiotics in order to prevent bacterial resistance.

Omits to talk about the side-effects of the drugs.

Upside of the treatment:

1. The parents are assured of being in the hands of a confident and knowledgeable doctor, with excellent patient management techniques. They feel safe
2. The doctor has recorded the data to support the treatment

Downside of the treatment:

1. The status of bacterial flora prior to illness is not known. The patient may have been harbouring the same bacteria in a state of good health. In that case, other factors like environmental changes, patient's constitution and the state of immunity may have had a significant role to play in the onset of disease
2. Till the culture/sensitivity results are available, it is a palliative (suppressive) treatment
3. In practice, culture/sensitivity tests are not routinely practised, so the practitioner resorts to the use of the latest anti-inflammatory and antibiotic drugs, whose side-effects could be significant. Sometimes, the microbes may not be sensitive to the chosen drug
4. Main treatment is directed against the microbes, which adapt easily to the changed environment, leading to drug resistance
5. The child may start suffering from recurrent throat infections. He is well only while the treatment continues
6. He is fast losing health, his appetite is poor, has loss of weight and is irritable. His immunity goes down. He may become sensitive to anti-inflammatory drugs which could lead to analgesic nephropathy causing renal failure
7. The parents are genuinely worried with the enormity of adversities. They impose lots of dietary and playing restrictions on the child. The child gets depressed. He becomes a potential candidate for the development of non-Hodgkin's lymphoma
8. Cost of the treatment is high

Homeopathic system of medicine

The conscientious homeopath takes a similar meticulous history, notes additional points in the history and clinical examination, which are relevant to remedy selection. A few examples:

1. Robust child, had gone for a picnic the previous day, played lots of games, had lots of ice cream and cold drinks. On examination, his face is flushed, skin dry, head hot and cold extremities, he has fear of ghosts and is comfortable with two pillows. The throat is glazed, congested and tonsils are enlarged.

Prescription: Bell. 30c, one dose three times a day.

The fever and pain in the throat are much better within 24–48 hours. Patient is well.

For frequent episodes, a constitutional medicine (*Calc.*), based on history is added.

2. Child had been depressed for the last few days because of the death of his pet dog. The pain in the throat was less while eating, more when not swallowing.

Prescription: Ign. 200c.

Patient has responded beautifully.

If the symptoms continue, a dose of *Nat-m. 200c* is added.

3. Child has been shivering and sweating the whole night, feeling very weak, pains in the entire neck extending to ears and chest, profuse secretions from nose and throat. Examination of the throat reveals

bluish-red swelling of tonsils, tongue is large, thick, with yellowish coating more in the posterior part.

Prescription: Merc-i-r. 200c

There is an amazing response to the medicine.

For recurrent episodes, suitable constitutional treatment is planned.

Upside:

1. Curative treatment starts with the first dose. Patient is well in a short time
2. No anxiety build-ups, no restrictions imposed on the child
3. No side-effects
4. There is no drug resistance as the treatment is not directed against the microbes

Downside:

1. Causative organism not known
2. It is presumed that the cause of the disease is annihilated with the cure. It is not recorded/tested
3. No auxiliary treatment prescribed; it is presumed that it has been taken care of
4. No patient management facilities available, which leads to lack of confidence in the physician and/or the system

This comparison helped me to decide that homeopathy was more suitable for the general practice of medicine, particularly with my background. I would keep transparent records of why and how a medicine would be selected, progress of the patient, timely investigations and referrals to suitable specialists.

Perhaps, the last straw was because of an incident that took place in the year 1995. Our family business was a construction company run by my husband and son. The entire staff of the company was used to taking homeopathic/allopathic treatment from me. My son was doing the interiors of a shop for his cousin in Chandigarh and had taken the entire staff from Delhi. The head supervisor (Mr P) was made to stay in the guest room on the ground floor of their home. The family rooms were on the first floor. At the turn of season, most of the crew fell sick with flu in varying degrees of severity. All were promptly well taken care of with allopathic medicines as my sister-in-law was a senior professor at PGI, Chandigarh. My brother-in-law, also a medical doctor, was very particular and took personal care of each one of them. One morning, while coming down the stairs, he overheard Mr P shouting at his son, who had just returned from Delhi, 'You fool, you went to Delhi and haven't brought medicine from Madam. Don't you see how we are all suffering here?' My brother-in-law was stunned and remained in shock for few days. He told me that the entire PGI (metaphorically) was at the command of the staff and yet they wanted homeopathy.

These experiences continued for twenty-two years. In the beginning, the prescriptions were mainly of allopathy. Homeopathy was tried in viral infections, where one had no specific treatment. As soon as the discharges turned thick and yellow, indicating a secondary bacterial infection as per my training, a suitable antibiotic was prescribed. It was also tried in diseases where the management was mainly empirical and where a large number of medicines was needed in management of diseases, such as diabetes or hypertension. Gradually and progressively, my knowledge of homeopathy and its application in clinical conditions increased. In the treatment of diabetes, hypertension and arthritis, the main medicine would be allopathic; associated symptoms like dyspepsia, insomnia and pains would be treated with homeopathy. This approach increased patient compliance, reduced morbidity and cost of treatment. I would give two prescriptions, one of allopathy and the other of homeopathy. All this added to my popularity as a clinician and I became known as a 'two prescriptions' doctor.

Progressively, the number of homeopathic prescriptions outgrew those of allopathy. I felt uncomfortable dispensing homeopathy as an allopath. I also realized homeopathy had become a system of beliefs for me. After much soul-searching, and many sleepless nights, I decided to take the MF (Hom) examination in the year 1997–98. I was already an associate member but with this I would become a member of the Faculty of Homeopathy, London, UK.

With the MF (Hom), I had gained expertise in treating the disease, but lost the privilege of being called a medical doctor. Validation for the path I chose came to me in two ways: through the patients I treated, and the recognition I received for my work.

PART TWO

Tryst with Homeopathy as a Homeopath

Eight

Decision to Restrict Medical Practice to Homeopathy

Clearing the MF (Hom) examination proved to be a milestone, the turning point in my life. I realized that my interest was not in the lucrative practice of medicine, but in the research and development of a safe, cost-effective and gentler therapeutic system, which gave reproducible results. Soon, opportunities came my way. First was a research project for the Homeopathy Medical College regarding the usefulness of homeopathy in the management of tuberculosis (TB) disease. The second opportunity came in 2008. It was an invitation to join a tertiary care multispeciality hospital, as a homeopath, and start an alternate medicine department. The facility which started as Pushpanjali Crosslay Hospital, Vaishali, Ghaziabad, is now known as Max Super Speciality Hospital, Vaishali. This was a golden chance for me to integrate homeopathy with allopathy.

Post this, I decided to restrict my medical practice to just homeopathy. This self-imposed restriction came in the wake of my desire to see how much could be achieved with only homeopathy. Successful cases had increased my confidence in the Similia principle, so much so that if I did not get results with homeopathy, I would blame my lack of knowledge rather than the therapeutic system.

The new protocol of my practice was that henceforth, I would prescribe only homeopathic medicines. If a patient was already on allopathic drugs, he/she would be asked to continue the same but I would explain that homeopathy would be added as a complementary treatment. That person was advised to continue with the treating physician because of the need and benefit of an integrated approach. Among other therapies to integrate homeopathy with, my preference would be for allopathy, as it was the mainstream mode of therapy, with excellent patient management facilities. A patient with multimorbidities would need treatment with procedures more than drugs, hence, it was prudent to be under the care of an allopath having hospital facilities. Since I had no knowledge of Ayurveda, I would refrain from combining homeopathy with Ayurveda. I considered physiotherapy, laboratory investigations, nutrition and dietary supplements as part of the general management of a patient and could be combined with any therapy.

Nine

Of Challenges and Learnings

As I stepped onto the road less travelled, the enormity of my decision hit me. From being an allopathic doctor, I had evolved into being a 'two prescriptions' doctor. Now, here I was, back to again being a single prescription doctor; this time, in the avatar of a homeopathic doctor. Only.

The first, and recurring, challenge I faced was when patients, sometimes, said that after a consultation with me, they had also consulted a 'medical' doctor. It seemed as if to them homeopathy was not medicine. As a 'two prescriptions' doctor, the addition of homeopathy to allopathy had improved my results vis-à-vis other general practitioners. Now, with only homeopathy, I had to get results which were as good or better than with allopathy to earn the trust of the naysayers. It was an uncharted path, full of blocks and crossroads, yet mentally stimulating and exciting. I knew I had my work cut out for me, but the silver lining was that that I didn't have to bring home the bacon.

Another challenge, discovered in the course of reading homeopathic texts, was that there were as many ways of prescribing as the number of books. In the last 250 years there had been many successful practitioners of homeopathy, who had chronicled their experiences in the form of books. Each one had felt confident of his/her method. It was all very confusing but, undaunted, I experimented with various methods and learned that what worked best for me was to have evidence-based reproducible results.

This experimentation and learning have continued for over four decades. Each patient has been examined and treated with a single thought: of both marking the boundaries of, and also learning the scope of, homeopathy. The raison d'être of the practice has been to find out what works for a patient and not, as described in the books of allopathy, for the disease. Epidemics have been a great learning experience: people of the same geographical area, climate and season have reacted with different intensities to the same microbe. The reaction has been subject to each person's state of vitality at that point in time. This state of vitality varies with the past and present mental and physical experiences and nutritional status of the person. Also, people of different geographical areas have differed with respect to the intensity and presentation of the disease. Hence, though the trigger has been the same 'microbe', and the main symptoms of the disease common, the ultimate combination of symptoms have differed in different people. However, there have been some clusters sharing the same set of medicines.

Another learning has been the understanding that people differ in their perception of a disease and its therapy. Some are die-hard believers of homeopathy, to the extent that it is difficult to persuade them to opt for allopathy, though that may be the right treatment for them at that point in time and stage of disease and vice versa. Experience has shown me that a person needs different therapies at different stages of the same disease. A nutrient deficiency can be addressed by a proper nutrition supplement; a sedentary habit by exercise and yoga. If the disease is functional, with many symptoms and normal investigations, homeopathy is the answer. A disease at an advanced stage, with structural changes, needs to be treated with allopathy. Sometimes, the disease is complicated, needing more than one therapy at the same time. A clinician has to be broad-minded and advise in the best interest of the patient.

Ten

Setting My Own Pattern

Concomitant to my advancement in medical practice, my prescriptions also advanced from a single medicine to multiple medicines. Experiences in formulating a regime for tuberculosis (TB) have taught me to formulate medicines, targeting a disease at multiple levels simultaneously, with the sole idea to bring about a cure in as short a time as possible. In this endeavour, I followed not the books, but my own intuition and logic. As an example: I was treating my thirty-six-year-old nephew for asthma. My analysis indicated *Puls.* for wheezing, which according to the books I had read, is a medicine for females. I was in a dilemma as to its usefulness in a male. After much thought, I examined his chest, gave one dose of *Puls.*, and asked him to wait in the clinic and inform me of any change, for better or worse, in wheezing. Almost immediately, he said that his wheezing had improved. Not believing him, I examined the chest again and found the wheezing sounds had actually reduced. Thereafter, gender bias was a low priority in my selection of medicine.

Each prescription, the first and subsequent one, was evaluated afresh with the help of *Repertory* and *Materia*

Medica. It was an effective method, though, sometimes contrary according to standard guidelines, which were: use of a single medicine, do not repeat the dose till the action of the previous medicine is complete. This dictum, laid out by the founder of homeopathy, Dr Christian Friedrich Samuel Hahnemann, was effective in simple, straightforward single diseases, but failed to produce the desired results in multifocal cases. For example, in the case of an elderly friend, who had sustained spinal injuries in a roadside fall out of a car, and where the muscles, ligament, tendons, nerves and bones were equally involved, I was in a dilemma as to which medicine was to be used first and for what duration. *Arnica* is for muscle injury, *Rhus tox* for ligaments and tendons. *Hypericum* for nerves, *Symphytum* for bones and *Ledum* for punctured wounds. All the parts of the body were equally important for the well-being of the patient. My logic guided me to give all medicines simultaneously. My friend, also a physician, accepted the homeopathic medicines reluctantly, but after a few days said, 'We don't see such quick results with allopathy.'

With time, I realized that for an effective prescription, addressing the presenting symptom/complaint, the timeline of the disease and underlying pathology simultaneously was most important. If all parameters were met with one medicine, the effect was magical. Otherwise, a combination of medicines, which complement each other, was needed with the presenting complaint present in all, maybe in various grades of intensity. I found *Repertory* helpful in formulating this prescription. Gradually, I stopped prescribing on a single symptom.

If there's any message from my work, it is that ultimately I dared to be different. I wanted to set my own pattern and to differ from both allopathy and homeopathy. Different from allopathy by using drugs diluted to an inconceivable extent, and from homeopathy by using multiple medicines at the same time. I soon realized that my allopath friends did not mind, as long as the results were coming. My homeopath friends kept quiet, while the patients, the most important people, were happy.

In the following pages, I have described some of my experiments and experiences.

Eleven

Experiments and Experiences

Single medicine versus multiple medicines

Treating a single disease was easy and rewarding. Protruding piles in a young woman, complaining of backache post-delivery, was cured within a week with *Kali-c.* An uncomfortable sensation of something stuck behind the sternum, making breathing difficult, was alleviated with *Abies-n.* Severe acute pain, felt in the centre of the chest after a hearty meal, without sweating or change in blood pressure, was cured with a couple of doses of *Nux-v.*, saving the patient a hospital visit.

But, piles of long duration in a patient, also suffering from chronic acidity and hypertension, did not get cured so easily. He needed a weekly dose of *Sulph.*, followed by *Nux-v.* (one of the options for piles), for a longer period. There were patients who suffered from dyspepsia, bloating and constipation and had tried many treatments, including single doses of homeopathy but without success, whereas a combination of *Lyc.* and *Carb-v.*, for a longer period, had a remarkable effect.

Closer home, during a surgical removal of the gall

bladder, I developed a painful tender swelling on my left wrist, the site where the needle for an intravenous drip had been inserted. I was instructed to use a thrombophob ointment locally. After five days of application, and a few doses of *Led.* (homeopathic medicine effective for punctured injury), the swelling was still hurting substantially. The surgeon added another antibiotic to the previous one and asked me to continue with the ointment. I had the option of having either two antibiotics or adding another homeopathic medicine. I chose the latter and took *Led.* and *Arn.* at two-hourly intervals, without waiting for the action of the previous dose to be over. By the end of the second day, there was no pain and the swelling and tenderness had reduced by half. A week later, the swelling too had disappeared.

There were cases of nasal block, associated with headache and other concomitants in various combinations and duration. I initially gave single doses of *Kali-bi.* to a patient with nasal block since the medicine symptoms and patient symptoms matched closely. He came after a month and said that after taking my medicine, he had developed his usual acute attack of a cold in moderate intensity and, since homeopathy was not effective in an acute phase (a common myth), he had taken allopathy but now wanted to continue with homeopathy. This set me thinking: could I treat both phases of the disease with only homeopathy? I took a detailed history of triggers for the onset and progress of acute symptoms, selected a suitable medicine, which was *Merc-i-r.*, and asked him to try it before taking allopathy. Next time, he managed with only an anti-allergic drug, no antibiotic; and subsequently with only homeopathy. Thereafter, such acute and chronic cases were effectively managed with two sets of medicine: one regular and the other for an acute episode. Both sets were according to a patient's symptoms, addressing the pathology of the disease and not according to the name, as per conventional medicine. For selection of medicines, I depended heavily on repertorization, followed by *Materia Medica*. So, for the same disease, though the main medicine would be the same, the combination could be different. Example: a patient, whose symptoms began with sneezing, and, on exposure to cold, increased at the sudden change of temperature, needed *Ars*. Another patient, who had a profuse thick discharge from nose and throat, needed *Puls.*; yet another patient who complained of frequent headaches, diagnosed as migraine, with scanty discharge and previous history of cold and cough, got *Sil.* along with *Kali-bi.*

Single medicine versus continued treatment

A medical student had suffered from pulmonary TB a year before, and was treated with Anti-tubercular Therapy (ATT) Cat III for six months. After being well for three months, he noticed a progressively increasing swelling on the right side of his neck, along with weakness, feverishness and loss of appetite. The Fine Needle Aspiration Cytology (FNAC) confirmed it to be of tubercular pathology. He consulted his physician, who advised him to wait and watch the progress of the disease, as he had completed the course of ATT only three months earlier. In the meantime, he took *Sil. 30c, 200c, Calc-p. 30c, Bac. 200c, Tuberculinum 200c* and *1M*, one after the another, in single doses at two to three weeks' interval on the advice of his senior teachers but without much effect. Last medicine was *Lyc. 200c*, taken a week before. My repertorization also indicated the same remedy. My prescription was a regime of three medicines: *Lyc. 200c* x 1 dose once a week, *Tub. 1M* x one dose once in 15 days and *Sil. 6D* three doses a day x 5 days a week. (*Tub. 1M* was selected as he had had it only a week before.) He had to take the medicines continually, without waiting for the action of the previous ones to be over.

After a month, the size of the lymph node started regressing, the offensive sweat reduced and the appetite improved. His treatment continued for five and a half months, at which point the lymph node was not palpable, nails had become normal and he had gained weight.

This case convinced me of the effectiveness of repetition of remedy at regular intervals in chronic diseases.

Single medicine versus frequent change in medicine

Should one give one constitutional medicine or treat the immediate presenting symptom bothering a multimorbid patient of advanced stage, was an enigma facing me. I had an elderly friend with multiple ailments, who, though under the care of senior physicians and on a handful of drugs, including antibiotic injections every day, was interested in homeopathic medicine. She would often ask for homeopathy for a symptom troubling her at that point in time. I decided one day to work on her constitutional medicine, and spent a whole night charting all her symptoms (I didn't have digital *Repertory* at that time). The homeopathic thought behind constitutional medicine is that if a medicine is chosen, encompassing all the symptoms of the disease and the patient's reactions to the environment and people, eating and sleeping habits, food preferences, that medicine will remove the underlying disease along with the symptoms. Such a treatment is curative in nature and, after a slight aggravation, the symptoms start disappearing in a particular order. I gave her a selected medicine with the advice that she should not take any other homeopathic medicine for a few days. Four hours later, she had taken three more medicines, besides the one I had given her: for redness of eyes, for right-side headache and for a nauseous feeling.

Realization dawned that a bothersome presenting complaint may not be due to the main disease but due to other causes: drug effect, dietetic error or psychosomatic reasons. In such a case, constitutional medicine would not be effective and the problem would be better treated with an indicated medicine, in medium to low dilutions on an as needed basis. Also, such a situation entailed a frequent change of medicine, depending on a change in symptoms.

Pills versus liquid preparation

Homeopathic medicines are commonly dispensed in pills made of cane sugar/milk sugar, medicated with the tincture of the indicated medicine and so look like the same 'sweet pills'. The tincture can also be taken as liquid after diluting it with water. In very sensitive people, olfaction has also been tried. I have preferred the pills form, both for the ease of dispensing for me and ease of carrying for the patient. In acute conditions however, my experience is that the liquid form is more effective.

One of my paediatric patients suffered from respiratory allergy. Her mother was handling the ailment with both conventional medicine and homeopathy. Once, at the age of nine, the child developed fever, followed by nose block and cough. The episode was managed with allopathy; the fever subsided but a dry wheezing cough continued to increase, in spite of three doses each of a bronchodilator and steroid inhalations. Homeopathic help was sought on the seventh day. I prescribed two medicines, one for dry cough and another for cough aggravated by coughing, along with a dose of *Phos.* in the morning in pills form. The allopathic inhalations continued, as the mother felt that the child could not do without them. By the third day the cough had increased and also the frequency of inhalations. Chest auscultation revealed no abnormality. I realized that the dry cough was partially due to frequent inhalations. There was a rubric (symptom) in *Repertory*: 'dyspnea felt in the nose with single medicine "*Puls.*"' This meant that the wheezing was because of constriction in the nose, not in the lungs, and the cough was due to dryness of the entire air passage. The prescription was changed to *Puls.* twice a day and a mix of three medicines (each medicine had its maximum action at different levels of the respiratory tract) in distilled water. The liquid medicine was to be taken frequently, with advice to reduce the inhalations. After five days, the cough had substantially reduced as also the frequency of inhalations to once a day.

Peculiar and rare symptoms

In homeopathic literature, great importance is laid on types of symptoms, particularly on peculiar and rare symptoms. Much later in my practice, I understood its importance. A lady doctor with a busy practice, came with the complaint of migraine, which began after the death of her husband. The episodes were frequent and moderately severe. Frequent use of pain-alleviating medicines had added gastric symptoms to her woes. She responded well to *Nat-m*. After a few weeks, she said that though the frequency and intensity of pain had reduced, she still needed pain-relieving drugs. *Ign.* was given as a complementary to *Nat-m.* which had no effect. On detailed interrogation, it was revealed that the headache was triggered when there were a few late nights in a row, and definitely when she was aroused from sleep. Repertorization indicated *Cocc.* which provided complete relief.

A forty-two-year-old lady was referred by the management of my hospital for body aches. The husband was carrying a fat file of her medical history. She was fair, plump and appeared to be mild and gentle. She suffered from peculiar pains in her entire body, especially the limbs, since she had moved to England from India. These were more prominent in the afternoon, incapacitating her totally, to the extent that she was unable to do any work. When her husband would come back from work in the evening, he would press (massage) her limbs, she would burp and get relief. In the *Repertory*, I found the rubric 'eructation on pressing the painful part' with a single medicine, *Borx*. This was prescribed twice a day, along with *Puls.* once in the morning (constitutional medicine). After a week of taking the two medicines, the patient was better by 80 per cent.

A sixty-one-year-old veterinary doctor came with the complaint of constant pain in his abdomen since eight months. The pain was associated with vomiting on attempting to swallow food when hungry. He would feel hungry but could not swallow food, because of intense nausea causing vomiting. He had lost six kilograms (kg) of weight. All attempts to diagnose the disease had failed and he was due for exploratory laparotomy (surgical opening of abdomen) the following fortnight. The rubric 'Nausea felt on swallowing' had the medicine *Merc-c.*, which made me examine his throat. I found an offensive odour, yellow post-nasal discharge, and thick dirty-white coating on the tongue. *Merc-c.* and *Kali-bi.* were prescribed. Within a week, he was eating normal food and the operation was cancelled.

Bedside medicine

There were times when a patient would be in a serious condition and no medicine would seem to be working, and I would be called upon to find if homeopathy had something. One day, when my associate Dr Priya Kapoor and I reached the hospital in the morning, we were told that a mutual friend was admitted in a serious condition. She was suffering from severe nausea and incessant vomiting since the previous evening. She had been taking drugs for high blood pressure and cervical pain and some drug reaction had led to this condition. In the hospital, various drugs had been tried in injectable form to control the nausea and vomiting, but nothing had been effective. Even an intravenous (IV) drip was not stable because of constant retching. It was a distressing sight to watch her in that condition. With no time to take a detailed history, we set about making a medicine for her condition. We selected four medicines indicated in nausea, vomiting and retching from various causes, put them in equal proportions in distilled water and asked the attendant to put two drops in the patient's mouth every half-an-hour. After two hours, the retching was less violent, the IV drip was stable and by evening she was able to hold sips of water. All the four medicines could treat constant and deathly nausea along with retching, with each medicine also having a different area of impacting with maximum effect. There was no time to fine-tune one medicine. End result was that our friend was saved from a serious condition.

One medicine for all

One of my homeopath friends was very fond of asking for tips for a specific medicine for a disease; similarly, an allopath friend wanted to know homeopathy 'Ram-baan' (specific medicine). Both wanted one medicine for one disease, which would work equally well in all cases.

This, to my understanding, is not possible. Different individuals react to the same stimulus in different ways, depending on their susceptibility and the sensitivity of the area of the body. Hence, each individual has a characteristic symptom complex, different from others, depending upon his/her environment and the state of the self-defence system. For example, people who have a tendency to overeat and are potential diabetics, could have a different combination of symptoms in homeopathic remedies such as:

Anacardium: Person has nervous dyspepsia and an empty feeling in the stomach. Eating temporarily relieves all discomfort, but the empty feeling comes back soon after eating. The person is constipated and desires to pass stool, but because of the effort required, the desire passes. Other symptoms are an irresistible desire to swear and curse; and a lack of self-confidence.

Nux vomica: Person has chronic dyspepsia, eats fast, desires fried food, is addicted to stimulants like tea, coffee, alcohol;

has gastric discomfort within a couple of hours after eating; has frequent, unsatisfactory, small stools; suffers from piles. He is a workaholic, dictatorial, arrogant and efficient.

Lycopodium: Person is prone to flatulence, few morsels cause bloating, yet overeats; suffers from acidity, heartburn; has constipation with effectual desire for bowel movement; piles; craves sweets and desires hot drinks. The person has a fear of speaking in public, but once he starts, does well; is an extrovert, is haughty, dictatorial towards those who can be controlled; and is timid and passive towards superiors.

Ignatia: Person has aversion to ordinary diet, longs for heavy indigestible food, is worse after drinking coffee; gets sour eructations, empty feeling in stomach which gets better by eating; has painful constriction of the anus after passing stool, suffers from suppressed grief, with long-drawn sighs and weeping spells, is hysterical with a tendency to spasms and headaches from tobacco smoke.

After studying the above medicines from *Materia Medica* in detail, it was clear that though all four had diabetes from overeating, they were different personalities and hence one medicine could not suit all.

Long-distance treatment

Sceptics pooh-pooh homeopathy and dismiss it as a placebo effect. What's more, the extreme dilution of the ingredients means the remedies are nothing more than sugar pills, they say. Some are even suspicious about the medicines being laced with steroids. This general impression is, to a large extent, due to the method of case taking, which is a prolonged sympathetic interaction. This section is not aimed at trying to 'prove' the validity of homeopathy to sceptics, who will never be convinced, but rather at providing an ad verbatim example of the clinical care and treatment homeopathy provides to patients. The case given below clearly showed me that the outcome from homeopathic drug intervention is quick, uncontaminated by steroids and without side-effects.

This is a case of online treatment of a child suffering from an allergic cough. The patient was the granddaughter of a friend, a pathologist in the USA. I had never met the patient. Both her parents were medical doctors, with the father a chest specialist. Below is the WhatsApp conversation between the grandmother, child's mother and doctor, that is me.

4th June 2019: My friend called from New Jersey, USA, asking if homeopathy could help in a chronic allergic cough. Her six-year-old granddaughter (Samara) was suffering from such a cough since the last three months. Allopathy, and cleaning the entire house for possible allergens, had not been effective. After getting some details from Samara's mother, I prescribed *Kali-bi. 30c* and *Phos. 30c*. The dose suggested was for liquid form. My friend had a box of homeopathic medicines, which she used for herself and others, from time to time on my advice.

5th June: Grandmother
Hi Kusumji, I have *Kali-bi. 30* as sugar pills and *Phos. 30D* as small tablets. So, instead of drops, I advised my daughter to give 4 pills of *Kali-bi.* (7 am and 7 pm) and 2 tablets of *Phos. 30D* (4 pm and 9 pm).

I hope I advised correctly?

She has also reduced the frequency of the Singulair and Ventolin inhaler to reduce the side-effects. Thanks.

6th June: Doctor

The dose is right. Do continue inhaler on as-needed basis.

6th June: Samara's mother to her mother (my friend)

Mummy, I got these medicines prescribed by you and have been using the following schedule.

Since they are not drops, Samara takes 2 pills of *Phos. 30 D* and 4 pills of *Kali-bi. 30c* for her doses.

6th June: Samara's mother (on a group she created for her mother and me called Samara's Cough)

On day 1 of this regimen, she had a very mild coughing bout in the evening, which lasted less than five minutes (instead of two hours). But she felt just as tired and complained of her throat hurting, just like it does in a prolonged cough.

On day 2 we decreased some of her meds (stopped Monteleukast, Cetrizine and changed Albuterol to SOS).

In the evening she did not have any cough, but had a slight post-nasal drip.

The previous night she had a rash on her cheeks that disappeared an hour later. It could have been from a new cream she used.

She also has a mild upset stomach for two to three days—that along with her fatigue made us stop the Monteleukast.

7th June: Grandmother

Hi Kusumji! SH has had no cough for two days but had some on the third day of starting homeopathic medicines.

7th June: Mother

Hello Aunty

Thank you so much for your advice regarding my daughter's cough.

She was previously on Foracort inhaler, Albuterol inhaler, Monteleukast and Cetrizine.

7th June: Doctor

Happy to know that Samara has shown some response. Please continue medicine in same dose for one week, along with nasal spray and inhaler on need basis.

In 2nd week if there is no/minimal cough, reduce medicine to once a day each. *Kali-bi.* 30c once at 4 pm, *Phos.* 30D once in morning

I will be out for 15 days. Any queries, ask by 8/6 evening, my time.

7th June: Grandmother

Thank you so much, Kusumji

20th June: Mother

Hi Aunty

SH has no cough and, except for red eyes, all other symptoms have subsided.

(End of WhatsApp conversation)

At this stage the chronic cough had vanished and allergy bouts were less frequent and milder.

Over time, I realized that for an effective prescription, addressing the presenting symptom/complaint, the timeline of the disease and underlined pathology simultaneously was most important. If all parameters were met with one medicine, the effect was magical; otherwise, a combination of medicines, which complemented each other was needed with the presenting symptom present in all, maybe in various grades of intensity. Use of *Repertory* was helpful in formulating this prescription. Progressively, I stopped prescribing on a single symptom.

PART THREE

Experiments In Childhood Diseases

Twelve

Homeopathy for Children: My Thoughts

Human beings are endowed with the power to heal themselves. The immune system of healthy people is able to keep many viruses, bacteria, fungi and other infectious agents at bay. This healing power is often greater for children than for older people. In a child, everything is young and bursting with energy, including the power of recovery. This is why most children get better on their own, with a bit of attention.

There are also children who are unable on their own to overcome certain ailments such as colds, ear infections, bronchitis, sore throat, sudden fever, violent pain, bouts of diarrhoea. These continue to reappear at sudden change in temperature, exposure to cold air, taking cold drinks, cold food or the slightest indiscretion in food. Homeopathic medicines stimulate the self-healing power of the body; curb the tendency to catch infections without implanting any significant side-effects.

Failure to address the ailments may lead to troubling fall-outs: the nights become long and punctured by the child's crying and discomfort. After a few years, these 'minor ailments' turn intolerable, parents are harassed by frequent visits to hospital, particularly at night. Sometimes, the parents' concern turns to anguish as the diminishing resistance of the child becomes so critical that survival becomes totally dependent on consumption of increasingly stronger antibiotics. This weakens the child further and parents get entangled in a vicious cycle. The addition of homeopathy at this stage breaks the vicious cycle, reduces the intake of antibiotics, the immune system becomes stronger, the frequency and intensity of infections decreases and the child's health improves, bringing peace and pleasure to the family.

In my practice of homeopathy, I have treated a large number of children, ranging from few-days'-old babies to adolescents. My experience of homeopathy in the diseases of infants and children is very positive. Most of the presenting symptoms in infants and young children may be associated with different illnesses and they often suffer from more than one illness; hence a syndromic approach is more effective. Homeopathy has the same approach: the disease is treated by careful evaluation of the presenting symptoms. One medicine can treat the symptoms of many diseases at the same time. Babies and children respond quickly to homeopathy; they love eating sweet pills, hence administration of medicine is no ordeal for the parents. Every time a child enters my clinic for the first time, he/she starts crying (defensive act), but then onwards, it's all smiles; it is not only for the sweetness of sugar pills, but also for the easing of painful symptoms. I am quite convinced about it, because the size of the smile is in direct proportion to the degree of wellness since the previous visit.

Given in the next few pages are a few of the many cases that benefited from my homeopathic treatment.

Thirteen

Childhood Diseases' Case Studies

Recurrent boils

My friend, a child specialist, asked me on 2 June 2009, whether homeopathy could treat recurrent boils in a fifteen-days'-old infant. His grandson was suffering from recurrent boils around the eyes, temples and navel. Local antiseptic applications were not helpful and he wanted to try homeopathy (or my knowledge) before antibiotics. It was a dilemma, regarding how to give and in what potency. After much deliberation, I got two small spray bottles, put two drops of *Sulph. 30c* in four ml of distilled water in one with a yellow cap and two drops of *Sil. 6c* in another bottle with a green cap. He was asked to spray the inside of the cheeks of the baby, once in the morning with the yellow cap bottle and twice a day with the green cap bottle. There were no boils after two days. The medicine continued for another day. No recurrence was noticed and no antibiotics needed.

Neonatal colic and nasal congestion

In the year 2008, my niece had her first baby. She was troubled by the baby's frequent crying from colicky pains and use of conventional anti-colic drops; she also wanted an alternate treatment for cold and cough. How to give medicine to a two-week-old baby was a dilemma. It would not be practical to prepare the medicine, one tablet to be dissolved in the mother's milk, with a crying baby at hand. So, I sent her the medicine in powder form and instructed her to dip the tip of a clean finger in the bottle of medicine and put the finger into the child's mouth. It was not as effective as allopathic colic drops in an acute phase; but over the next ten days, after doing this once a day, she felt that the intensity and frequency of colic had reduced.

For cold and cough, I mused that, 'though a newborn baby is homeothermic, his/her ability to stay warm may be easily overwhelmed by changes in environmental temperature, making him/her vulnerable to respiratory infections. Exposure to cold is inevitable with frequent change of nappies. *Ferr-p.* is indicated in the first stage of all inflammatory affections particularly chest trouble.' So, for cold and cough, I thought *Ferr-p.* 6D would be a good medicine and it would also help in improving the baby's haemoglobin.

This led me to make a preparation of equal portions of *Ferr-p.* 6D and *Mag-p.* 6D in powder form.

I advised my niece to give one full fingertip of this powder twice a day, without any symptoms, till the baby was three months old. The outcome was good, there was no severe colic or nasal congestion or feeding problem with the baby and the mother didn't have to suffer strict dietary restrictions.

This powder soon became popular in the extended family and with my regular patients. A few examples:

- Raghav came on 16 January 2015 for the regular treatment of his six-year-old daughter. He asked me whether there was any treatment for colic in a newborn baby in homeopathy. His second child had been born about two weeks ago, and was getting frequent pain in the abdomen from wind colic, which would get better by making her lie on her stomach. I prescribed powder of *Ferr-p.* 6D and *Mag-p.* 6D as one fingertip twice a day and *Coloc.* 30c, one pill dissolved in the mother's milk for acute pain. Feedback on 31 January 2015, was that *Coloc.* was needed for the first few days; after that the intensity of pain had lessened. He was advised to continue with the powder for three months.
- Final validation of its efficacy came in 2018, when my daughter had her second baby. Four years earlier, when she came home after delivery, the baby would be cranky every evening. Her husband was averse to giving any medicine to his child, more so homeopathy. After trying various things, he agreed to try my powder, when the baby was wailing but found it ineffective. On my request, it was given every morning and afternoon, without any symptom. Colic stopped after two to three days and so also the medicine; as the family was of the view that medicine is only taken in sickness. I firmly directed my daughter to be regular with the powder and the result was comfort, as comfortable as it can be with a newborn. So, in 2018, when they were in hospital for the second delivery, he told my daughter to get the powder for the baby, before they came home from the hospital.

- One of my patients who had been infected by the human immunodeficiency virus (HIV) had a baby after much effort and wait. She brought the baby to me at six weeks, in September 2019. He had a cough and chest congestion for two weeks. Chest congestion had improved with antibiotics, but the cough was troublesome. *Phos. 30c* and *Ip. 30* for one week were given for the cough, followed by *Ferr-p. 6D* and *Mag-p. 6D* powder. The baby had no respiratory complaint till four months of age.

Cranky and colicky children

I had gone to meet my brother-in-law's family; my niece was visiting with her nine-month-old baby. She was looking troubled and exhausted. The baby would start crying if she sat down; he just wanted to be walked while being carried in the lap. I gave him a dose of *Cham.* and after half-an-hour, both mother and son were sleeping.

I got a call from my son-in-law (RS) one afternoon that the seven-year-old son was howling with pain in the tummy. My daughter, who kept the homeopathic medicines, was not at home. From her kit, one dose of *Nux-v. 30c* was given but the child continued to howl. RS was a non-believer in homeopathy and my knowledge of prevailing anti-colic allopathic medicine was rusted, hence, it was decided to take him to the hospital. On a video call, I saw the child was bent double, pressing the tummy. He complained that the pain was coming in spurts. The right medicine was *Coloc.* It was not in the kit, so a person was rushed to the nearby homeo-pharmacy. After a dose of the medicine, the howling stopped and after two hours the child had a full meal followed by a hearty dinner in the evening. RS was left wondering whom to believe: the child or homeopathy.

Pruritis

I was treating a sixteen-year-old boy for recurrent episodes of tonsillitis. Antibiotics were helpful, but were unable to prevent the episodes. After a few months, the episodes lessened, so also the need of antibiotics. He asked me, whether homeopathy had treatment for bleeding piles. On affirmation, he brought his sister who had developed piles after her first delivery. When she felt an improvement in her condition, she asked if homeopathy could be given to babies as well. I assured her of its effectiveness in children. She talked about her sixteen-month-old baby, who had an itching all over the body for the last six months, but without any rash, or change in colour or texture of the skin. At that present time, the baby had been vomiting since the last five to six days. She usually passed pale yellow-coloured stools, two to three times a day, her appetite was poor, she had an aversion to milk, an increased thirst for water; loved eating soil and was in the habit of putting everything in her mouth.

I prescribed a constitutional medicine based on the indications: desires eating earth (indigestible thing), puts everything in her mouth. Next week, she was initially better and then itching started again. This time the medicine was prescribed on the indication: itching without eruption and light-coloured stools. Three weeks later, the itching was much better, but the child wanted to eat paint; this time the constitutional medicine was given once a week, followed by six days of medicine for itching. After three weeks, there was no itching, her appetite had improved, but the tendency to put everything in her mouth and eating indigestible things was still present. A weekly dose of constitutional medicine was given in higher potency. There were no complaints thereafter.

Observation: This case taught me that skin problems are the result of internal dyscrasia, better treated with internal medicine. Also, when constitutional medicine is followed by medicine based on local symptoms in lower potency, recovery is faster and lasting.

Delayed speech with chronic tonsillitis

An anxious elderly man requested me for an early appointment for his grandson. His son, a resident of Spain, was visiting India with his family. The grandparents were worried that in spite of good medical care in Spain, their grandson was not talking at the age of three years; he could only babble incoherent words. The entire family came for consultation on 4 March 2010. There was a history of recurrent attacks of tonsillitis since infancy, treated with antibiotics. Typically, an attack of moderate to high fever would come suddenly on slightest exposure to cold. He was an active, playful child, especially at night; but could turn violent and hurt others, particularly his mother. The child hardly slept at night; had a good appetite, sweated profusely on the head while sleeping. His other milestones were normal. Examination of the throat revealed hypertrophy of both tonsils, which were bright red in colour and enlarged, with mobile and tender submandibular cervical lymph nodes on both sides of the neck

I decided to base my prescription not on the symptom of defective and delayed speech but on the pathology of recurrent tonsillitis and the child's behaviour.

Prescription on 4 March 2010: Bell. 30c, one dose in the mornings, six days a week for sudden fever, excitable violent nature; *Sil. 6c* twice a day, six days a week for enlarged cervical lymph nodes; *Calc. 30c*, three doses once a week for profuse sweating on the head on sleeping; *Tub. 200c*, one dose once a month for recurrent tonsillitis; with the advice to treat acute episodes of fever locally with allopathy. The family was leaving for Spain in a few days. The medicine was given for two months, with advice to review after three weeks.

The patient's mother telephoned after three weeks to inform me that the child was better and had not suffered any acute attack of fever. She was advised to continue treatment till medicines lasted.

The grandparents were going to Spain on 10 May 2010 and wanted to carry medicine for seven to eight months. The feedback from the mother was that the child's health had improved. He had suffered from fever only once, which was treated with antibiotics leading to fast recovery; had started talking with hesitancy, which was accompanied by drooling of saliva from mouth. But he got excited on seeing people, was active and sleepless at night and could turn violent.

10 May 2010: Lach. 200c, two doses once a week was given for swelling of tonsils, excitement at night causing sleeplessness and difficult speech; *Sulph. 30c* was selected for swelling of tonsils and as a complementary medicine to *Lach.*; *Nux-v. 30c* was given for chilliness, aggravation from cold air and excitable nature; *Tub. 200c*, two doses once a month was for recurrent tonsillitis.

The mother gave a feedback on 9 December 2010 that the child had started talking, episodes of fever were few and short, sleep had improved, size of the cervical lymph nodes and violent behaviour had reduced. The complaint was excessive sweating on the head while going to sleep and pain in the ear. She wanted medicine for about two months, when they would be visiting India. The new prescription on 7 December 2010 was a regime of *Calc. 30c*; *Sil. 30c* and *Sulph. 200c*.

The parents and grandparents, along with the child, visited my clinic on 27 January 2011. His speech was normal, he was talking in full sentences, there was no pain in the ear or fever or sore throat, the sweating on the head was much reduced, cervical lymph nodes soft and small (less than 1 cm). The family wanted medicine for a further six months, to prevent recurrence of sore throat and pain in the ear. I suppressed a smile because that's what I had been treating the patient for right from the beginning, since I knew that the root cause was tonsillitis.

Observation: The patient was brought for the treatment of a symptom of delayed speech, but the treatment regime was based on the underlying cause, reached through symptoms of recurrent tonsillitis, effect of exposure to cold and behaviour. I had learned the importance of reaching the cause of the disease through symptoms; and also changing the prescription according to the change in presenting symptoms.

Atopic dermatitis

A pretty petite two-year-old baby would be so itchy that she would not stop scratching herself till bleeding ensued. She was born with a dry skin, but for the past one month, had developed red-coloured, round rough spots all over the body, with new spots appearing before the older ones healed. Her paediatrician and skin specialist had treated her with various local applications and antibiotics, without any significant improvement. The worried parents had gone to the city's senior-most paediatrician, a kind-hearted soul, who promptly referred the case to me.

I saw the patient, a sullen-faced, whiny child, on 12 July 2017. She had an unhealthy spotted dry skin with scratch marks all over the body. There were no other complaints. Two medicines: *Sulph.* and *Ars.* were given in low potency frequency, two times each, with *Graph.* as a weekly dose. For local application, parents were advised to continue with previously recommended lotions. Two weeks later, the old eruptions were drying, new ones were small and few, more near the bends of the knee and elbow joints. Another medicine was added to the regime, more suitable for eruptions near the bends of joints. On 18 August 2017, five weeks later, new lesions were absent and all lesions had dried up, but itching was prominent. BCH drops in the moisturizer for local application was added. (BCH drops are a combination of mother tinctures of *Berb-a.*, *Calen.* and *Ham.* mixed in equal proportion. This liquid is added to a suitable moisturizer in the proportion of one drop of this to one ml of moisturizer followed by succussion, resulting in a medicated moisturizer. I have found it to be effective and soothing in dry, rough skin and minor cuts and cracks.) The body was free of eruptions on 15 September 2017, but the skin was dry and itchy. The parents were advised to use less soap and moisturize the skin daily and often.

Observation: All the medicines were indicated and complementary. The combination led to a smooth and speedy recovery without aggravation.

Mundan ceremony

A three-year-old child was brought by his mother for the complaints of running nose and mild fever. He had been under my care since the age of four months and had a tendency to get attacks of a running nose, which would often develop into wheezing and a bad cough, which got worse at night on lying down, ending in vomiting. She was scared of this episode worsening into a wheezing attack, as the next day was the big function of his mundan (first haircutting ceremony), and she wanted some preventive medicine for him to remain well. I made a liquid preparation of two medicines, one for the bad effects of haircutting and another for running nose and wheezing, and advised the mother to give 5 ml every three hours. The child was well during the function and the mother was happy.

Observation: It was a new experience to know that homeopathy can be used as a preventive medicine.

Long-term management of recurrent infections and allergy

The hospital had been recently commissioned and one September morning in the year 2009, I went to say hello to the head of the pathology department. She was looking perturbed and tired. On enquiring, she told me that the previous night her granddaughter, a sixteen-month-old baby, was admitted in hospital for an attack of suffocative cough and wheezing. This was the third time in two weeks. Medicines were effective in aborting the attack but were unable to prevent it. On my suggestion, she agreed to try homeopathy. Next morning, the parents and the baby came for consultation. She was a delicate and irritable child, refusing to be touched. She had been suffering from colds and cough since birth, and was a poor eater. Lately the intensity of the rattling cough with wheezing had increased, particularly at night. She would wake up suddenly with a suffocating cough ending in vomiting, followed by refusal to eat/drink anything. It was distressing for the parents as she had to be rushed to hospital. *Puls.*, morning and evening, and *Ip.* before lunch and dinner was prescribed, with the advice to continue with ongoing treatment. Two weeks later, the symptoms decreased, appetite had improved and there were no night visits to hospital.

After the acute episode was handled effectively, the parents came for long-term treatment of allergy to milk and eggs and to raise her immunity. She was given a weekly dose of *Sulph.* along with morning doses of *Sil.* and *Ferr-p.*, twice a day on other days of the week.

Three weeks later, the patient reported a stuffy nose and a cough but no vomiting and she could be managed well at home. She was being nebulized with a bronchodilator drug every evening. As she was very irritable, she was prescribed *Nux-v.* twice a day, *Sulph.* and *Ferr-p.* were continued. After two weeks, she was off the nebulizer totally and was more interactive and cheerful.

She was doing fine with this treatment plan, but complained of a rattling cough with vomiting in November. *Ant-t.* along with *Ip.* given twice a day and one dose of *Puls.* at night for a few days along with nebulization once in the evening restored her health.

She was still allergic to milk and getting quite stubborn. *Calc.* as two doses once a week, and *Puls.*, morning dose six days of the week was all that she needed. Later, in the cold of December, she travelled to Goa where there was high humidity and did not need any nebulization. She was advised to continue with the same regime of medicines, even without symptoms.

In the last week of January, the patient complained of pain in the abdomen due to dentition. A few doses of *Mag-c.* removed the complaints and later she was again put on her regular treatment.

In March, she travelled to Vaishno Devi and developed a slight running nose and cough, but there was no wheezing. Her mother used the SOS (comprising *Ip.* + *Ant-t.*, given as emergency treatment) in the morning and at bedtime from fear of it developing into suffocating wheezing, and *Puls.* twice during the day. Within three days she was fine without any other medication.

In June 2010, her mother brought her though she was quite well. She had been taking a regime of weekly doses of *Calc. 30c* with six days of *Ferr-p.* The same treatment plan was continued in view of the changing season and her tendency for easy coryza. She was eating well and could tolerate milk and eggs also. The visits to the emergency room were a thing of the past and she was a healthy child who continued to grow well.

Observation: The transformation of a sick and irritable child into a healthy blossoming child and distressed parenting to happy parenting was a reward worth becoming a homeopath.

Long-time management of recurrent infections

Prabhat, a three-and-a-half-year-old boy, was brought to my clinic by his grandfather on 27 May 2002 for complaints of recurrent fever with sore throat, abdominal pain with loose stools. Every episode was effectively treated with conventional medicine, but of late, the frequency of illness had increased, hence the homeopathic consultation to increase the immunity. The illness began with a running nose, followed by pain in the throat and rapid rise in temperature, usually after exposure to cold air/drinks. Eating fried food and too many chocolates caused pain in the abdomen, followed by frequent stools and fever. He sweated profusely on his head while sleeping and was very shy. The examination revealed a large tongue with indented margins and a thick dirty-white coating, more at the back of the tongue; both tonsils were hypertrophied and congested. The child was fond of chocolates, butter and milk. His mother was a medical doctor, presently staying in a hostel for her studies, which resulting in too much pampering. There was a family history of respiratory allergy in the mother and paternal uncle.

Bell., three doses a day was prescribed for abdomen pain on 27 May 2002. Three days later, the pain was less but stools were frequent. I gave *Calc.*, three doses once a week, for profuse sweating on head, and *Merc-i-r.*, one dose a day, for frequent stools. The patient came back after about a month on 3 July 2002. His runny nose had stopped, weight had increased, sweat on the head was reduced and he had mild fever for one day only. The grandfather wanted medicine for the appearance of white spots (light-coloured) on the face, arms and abdomen of the child, aggravated after eating cottage cheese. *Sep. 200c* for white spots in the child was prescribed. Patient had a runny nose and cough after three days, which were treated effectively with a daily dose of *Merc-i-r.* Paroxysmal cough was more at night, and it did not respond to *Kali-bi. Sep.* was repeated after three weeks again on 29 July 2002. It was followed by an acute attack of cold, cough and fever. This was treated with conventional medicine and antibiotics. *Carb-v.* was prescribed for weakness felt after antibiotics. Three doses of *Psor.* were given as intercurrent antipsoric treatment on 21 August 2002. Thereafter, for the next three months, the patient was treated with weekly doses of *Hep. Puls.* for runny nose, and *Spong.* for dry cough. He was well, except for one mild attack of fever managed with only homeopathy. On 13 January 2003, he developed moderate fever with nasal discharge and frequent cough with easy expectoration, effectively treated with *Hep.*, one dose in morning, and *Merc-i-r.* two-three times a day. Now, the grandfather asked for homeopathic medicine for stammering, if any. Same regime was continued for the next three months and the patient did not need any antibiotics. On 26 March 2003, the complaint of dry, itchy patches on the skin, not responding to any anti-allergic drug and antibiotic, improved remarkably with weekly doses of *Kali-bi.* and *Sil.* Thereafter, treatment with *Sil.*, one dose a day, kept the patient well for the next eight months. On 2 December 2003, he was given three doses of *Calc. 30c* for excessive sweat on the head. Treatment continued for a further eight years with weekly doses of *Sil.*, *Puls.* and *Kali-bi.* (for blocked nose). Excessive sweating on the head and white patches on the skin in the year 2006 responded well to *Calc.*

Observation: The family was very happy with the homeopathic treatment, though they had no faith in the system. The child was off frequent use of anti-allergic drugs and antibiotics and thriving. It was a great learning for me too. *Sep.* was perhaps the wrong choice for this patient, though indicated in 'light-coloured spots in a child'; I had treated two boys with the same complaint successfully at that point in time, hence the prescription. But generalization does work in homeopathy; this boy was a *Calc.* patient. Also, use of *Kali-bi.* in 2002 was wrong; it wasn't even effective and on hindsight *Phos.* was more indicated.

There are many more cases, and while the diseases, symptoms and treatment differ in almost each one, what is common is the satisfaction I have got from being able to give relief to both the babies and their parents. The ability to share my knowledge of homeopathy to positively impact a young person's health has definitely been a cause of joy in my career.

PART FOUR

Experiments In Urinary Complaints

Fourteen

Integration of Two Systems for Urinary Complaints

Urination is the body's way of getting rid of excess water as well as wastes. While this is an important function for survival, urinating too frequently can interfere with a person's quality of life. Each person may pee a different number of times per day, depending on how much one drinks and how well that person's kidneys work. The frequency is near constant for one individual in health. While one is occasionally likely to go more frequently than that, a daily change in frequency of peeing, especially during the night, waking one from sleep, may signal a concern for too-frequent urination. This calls for a regular macroscopic and microscopic examination of morning samples of urine. This simple and easy-to-perform test imparts a wealth of information about the functioning of the urinary system, which comprises two kidneys, two ureters, one urinary bladder and a urethra.

Increased urination with normal urine examination and no other symptoms could be due to: drinking too many drinks causing excess caffeine intake through coffee, tea, and certain soft drinks; generalized obesity placing extra pressure on the bladder; abdominal obesity (potbelly) leading to weakness of pelvic muscles; menopause from low oestrogen levels, when chilled or occupied; and old age. Presence of sugar in urine indicates undiagnosed diabetes, which should be promptly attended to. Presence of pus cells and a positive leucocyte esterase is indicative of infection anywhere in the urinary tract; if it is in the kidney, it is called pyelonephritis; in the bladder, cystitis; and in the urethra, urethritis; which should be effectively dealt with. Leaving it untreated can lead to serious problems in the future, like hypertension, renal failure.

Women tend to get urinary tract infections (UTI) more often because their urethra is shorter and closer to the anus than in men. Because of this, women are more likely to get an infection after sexual activity or when using a diaphragm for birth control. These cause serious discomfort to women and have a high impact on ambulatory healthcare costs, through outpatient visits, diagnostic tests and prescriptions. About 50 to 60 per cent of women have at least one episode of cystitis after puberty. In majority of cases, the first episode coincides with the beginning of sexual intercourse. Recurrent urinary tract infection (R-UTI) is defined as three or more episodes in twelve months or two or more episodes in six months. Cystitis after intercourse (post-coital cystitis [PCC]) accounts for 60 per cent of recurrent cystitis. Most physicians treat R-UTIs with multiple courses of antibiotics, often leading to antibiotic resistance. The high prevalence of R-UTIs and the worsening of the frequency pattern of PCC clearly indicate that this bacteria-oriented approach, although evidence-based medicine (EBM) supported, in the long-term is ineffective for many women. It has been observed that antibiotic resistance increases the relapse rate in UTIs. What we need is effective alternatives, in particular for antibiotics.

Antibiotics are medicines used to prevent and treat bacterial infections. Resistance to antibiotics occurs when bacteria change their response to the use of these medicines. Bacteria, not humans or animals, become antibiotic-resistant. These resistant bacteria are harder to treat, leading to higher medical costs, prolonged hospital stays and increased mortality.

Results of a World Health Organization (WHO) survey carried out across twenty-two high- and low-income countries between March 2016 and July 2017 revealed antibiotic resistance to a number of serious bacterial infections. WHO spokesman Christian Lindmeier said the survey's findings raised many red flags among health professionals who admitted, it was 'one of the biggest threats to global public health'.

The world urgently needs to change the way it prescribes and uses antibiotics. A total reliance on only antibiotics has been an easy and one-sided approach. A change in behaviour and recognizing the importance of the self-defence mechanisms (SDM) of living beings is important in combating antibiotic resistance. Without these, it will remain a major threat, even if new medicines are developed.

In treating a disease with allopathy, the whole attention is on the immediate external cause, for example, microbes. SDM is taken for granted as a constant factor, while it waxes and wanes. When it is low, one is more prone to disease and the treatment is difficult and prolonged. While homeopathy seems to affect SDM and makes it stronger, antibiotics act and reduce the microbial load. Homeopathy and allopathy are both complementary to each other and integration of the two systems can be beneficial in the treatment and prevention of antibiotic resistance.

Following are a few examples of urinary complaints, effectively managed with only homeopathy, or in combination with allopathy, in multimorbid patients.

Fifteen

Management of Urinary Complaints

Urinary tract infection with bronchial asthma

One Saturday afternoon, my associate, forty-one years old, went for an outing to a mall. By 8 pm, she had developed acute discomfort in her lower abdomen, along with increased frequency of urination. She took *Canth. 200c* in liquid form every one hour till she fell asleep, then every three hours when she woke up for urination. This dosage continued the next day. Her symptoms reduced by 80 per cent for a few hours in the afternoon, but returned to previous intensity by the evening. She was an asthmatic, taking steroids and bronchodilators as inhalers and had a cough, with easy and copious expectoration at that time. Her symptoms were repertorized on Monday morning, taking into consideration urinary as well as bronchial symptoms. The symptoms were: burning pain in the urethra before, during and after urination, sore pain in the urethra, inflammation of the bladder; asthmatic respiration, copious and easy expectoration. *Puls. 30c*, one dose every two hours was prescribed as it had the highest scoring points. The patient took additional two doses of *Canth. 200c* as she was apprehensive of pain. The urine examination showed a full field of pus cells. Next day, pain and frequency of urination was reduced by half, urine microscopic examination showed a reduced number of pus cells. Mid-stream urine sample was given for culture and sensitivity. It was positive for *Klebsiella* (a type of bacteria) sensitive to most antibiotics. Since there was marked reduction every day in symptoms and of pus cells in urine, it was decided to continue with the same homeopathic treatment and not switch to antibiotics, though strongly advised by her conventional medical physician. Urine routine and culture examination was repeated after eight days. The result showed pus cells were 3–4/hpf and culture was sterile. A repeat examination after three months showed the same results.

Observation: This case was a great learning for me. It taught me the meaning and importance of totality of symptoms. The patient had an acute UTI, for which *Canth.* is a good medicine, but it was not the correct similimum for the patient, as this patient was also suffering from acute respiratory infection at that point in time. When considering only urinary symptoms, *Canth.* was indicated, but its effect was not lasting. *Puls.* covered both urinary and respiratory symptoms, leading to a fast and lasting cure. This was a marked deviation from the allopathic way of treating disease. It also taught me that homeopathy can be effective in acute infections and has rapid action.

Recurrent prostatitis

Manmohan Singh, a seventy-one-year-old medical doctor, came on 2 June 2009 with the complaint of pyuria of three years' duration; after prostatectomy for an enlarged prostate. He had increased frequency of urination, which was troublesome. The urine microscopic examination showed 10–15 pus cells/hpf, but the urine culture test was always negative. Since he was in frequent contact with TB patients, the possibility of TB was being thought of, but he was averse to taking conventional ATT. *Lyc. 200c* three times a day for six days a week, followed by *Thuj. 1M* three doses on the seventh day was prescribed for two weeks. This prescription was on the basis of a desire for warm drinks (tea), frequent urination, pyuria and inflammation of the prostate gland. Two weeks later, the frequency of urination and the pus cells in urine had reduced to 0–1/hpf. The same medicine was repeated for another two weeks.

Observation: The most common clinical diagnosis for presence of urinary symptoms and pus cells in urine with negative urine culture for aerobic bacteria is TB. The patient may have had some uncommon anaerobic infection or lowered immunity from prolonged suffering which led to continued symptoms. Treatment with homeopathy led to subjective and objective improvement.

Urethral stricture

Arjun Kumar, a fifty-nine-year-old medical doctor, came on 1 May 2018 with the complaint of urethral stricture from latex allergy due to insertion of Foley's catheter during a prostectomy operation. His acute burning pain lasted for thirty minutes after urination and he had to undergo mechanical dilation every day, which was extremely painful. There was a history of UTI with *E. coli.* twenty days earlier, treated with *Clem. 30c, Sil. 6D* and *Calc-f.*, twenty days ago. Now *6D. Sulph. 30c* twice a day at 6 am and 4 pm, *Merc-c.*

30 twice a day at 8 am and 8 pm, *Sil. 6D* three times a day at 11 am, 3 pm and 10 pm was prescribed.

On 12 May 2018, the procedure of dilatation was less painful and it was reduced to alternate days. Burning pain during urination was also less. The patient complained of left-sided ringworm-like lesions in the groin, at the knee joint and nape of the neck. Prescription was changed to *Sulph. 30c*, one dose in morning, *Sep. 30c* one dose in evening, *Thuj. 200c*, three doses once a week on Sunday; *Merc-c. 30c, Sil. 6D* continued as before. Treatment was repeated on 22 May 2018 as dilatation was needed after every three days, with lesser pain and no burning during urination. On 31 May 2018, dilatation was needed after six days, was painless, and all skin lesions gone except for those on the neck.

Observation: Multiple medicines were prescribed simultaneously, each targeting some part of pathology. *Sulph.* was for allergy to latex of the catheter, inflammation and stricture of the urethra, *Merc-c.* for inflammation, ulceration of meatus and pain during urination, *Sil.* for stricture of the urethra, *Sep.* for stricture and skin lesions. Each medicine had a different combination with inflammation of the urethra. The patient was in acute distress and the regime led to fast recovery.

Multimorbid drug-resistant urinary tract infection (UTI)

A seventy-four-year-old lady, wife of a homeopath, sought homeopathic treatment for culture positive drug-resistant UTI on 30 January 2015. She had recurrent UTI for over two decades, along with diabetes, cystocele and prolapsed uterus. These were also the maintaining cause of recurrence. Diabetes was of twenty years' duration, which was managed with oral hypoglycemic (sugar lowering) drugs with average control of blood sugar levels. The advice to switch to injectable insulin preparation by the treating endocrinologist had not been complied with. She also had complete prolapse of the urinary bladder (grade III cystocele) and uterus, but the surgical treatment was ignored for fear of complications, particularly in the presence of diabetes. With such co-morbidities, she was very particular about UTI and had urine culture done at regular intervals. Being a meticulous person, she had kept all records, filed in chronological order. Regular use of antibiotics for prophylaxis and cure had kept the infection under control till she developed infection with an unusual bacterium *Serratia marcescens*, needing use of strong antibiotics, causing intolerable adverse drug effects and subsequently became resistant to them.

Her homeopath husband had been treating her with single doses of homeopathy without perceptible improvement. This time also, he gave medicines directed at only urinary symptoms, without taking into account prolapse and diabetes. The treatment was ineffective as it was not holistic. This unnerved the patient, hence the consultation. Our regime incorporated all the pathology, leading to not only recovery from infection, but also improvement in degree of diabetes and prolapse.

Another interesting observation was the changing pattern of the urine culture reports. Within the first six weeks of treatment with only homeopathy, there was a marked improvement in symptoms and the infection with *Serratia marcescens* became responsive to antibiotics, which was a great mental relief to the patient; subsequently, the urine culture report was negative, indicating absence of infection. Whenever there was a lapse in taking medicine for about a week, the urine would become turbid and culture positive. As the patient found allopathy more convenient, she would switch to antibiotics. First time there would be quick response, making her happy; but to her dismay, there would be an earlier recurrence, with bacteria becoming drug-resistant without homeopathy. She realized that regular use of homeopathy brought about increased sensitivity to antibiotics, while every course of antibiotics led to drug-resistance. Thereafter she was regular with homeopathy, until October 2017, with much reduced recurrence and no drug-resistance. At this point, she felt that she could manage herself with increased water intake and cranberry supplements and discontinued treatment. (For more details see article: Chand, Kusum S., Kapoor, P. 'Two Case Reports of Integrated Management of Antibiotic Resistant Urinary Tract Infection', *Homeopathy,* 2020, 109 [02]): 92–106.

Observation: Regular use of a homeopathic regime, incorporating all the pathology, led to recovery not only from infection, but also improvement in the degree of diabetes and prolapse. Another interesting observation was that consistent use of homeopathy brought about increased sensitivity to antibiotics while every antibiotics caused drug-resistance.

Post-coital cystitis

Lata Singh, a forty-five-year-old lady, came for consultation on 10 October 2017, with the complaint of recurrent episodes of *E. coli* culture positive UTI of eighteen years' duration. She had been on antibiotics, both for prophylaxis as well as for an acute episode, without any long-term benefit. There was post-coital aggravation, and her post-coital burning was a constant nagging feature. At the time of consultation, she had been on injection *Amikacin*® for a week as her infection was resistant to most other drugs.

Her response to two weeks of a homeopathy regime was effective. It comprised *Sep. 200c*, one dose in the evening, two doses a day of *Canth. 30c* for six days of the week, followed by three doses of *Staph. 1M* on the seventh day every week. *Sep.* was given for chronic cystitis, *Canth.* for burning during urination, and *Staph.* for post-coital aggravation. She was symptom-free for four weeks without treatment. On 28 December 2017, the post-coital burning recurred (urine culture not done), so she wanted to be on regular homeopathic medication. The same regimen was continued for the next two months, when she remained symptom-free and the urine was sterile. Considering the remarkable response of the patient, it was decided to reduce the medication to weekly doses of *Sep. 200c* and *Staph. 1M*; *Canth. 30c* was to be added on the appearance of symptoms. After two months, on 28 April 2018, as there was no relapse she was taken off the treatment on the adage 'no symptoms, no disease'.

The patient was asymptomatic for about three months without any treatment. On 9 August 2018 she came with the complaints of increased frequency and burning during urination since three to four days. Initial prescription comprising *Sep. 200c, Canth. 30c* and *Staph. 1M* was repeated; both urine microscopic as well as culture examination, were advised. She returned only after about three weeks. Urine microscopic examination had shown 10 WBC/hpf and culture was positive for *Citrobacter koseri* 10^5 *cfu/ml*. This time she had needed antibiotics for two weeks as treatment for the acute episode. For prevention of a relapse, she was advised *Lyc. 200c, Berb. 30c* and *Sil. 30c* each, two doses a day for two weeks. *Lyc.* was given for chronic cystitis, *Berb.* for acute as well as chronic cystitis, and *Sil.* for the tendency to recurrent inflammation. She did not visit the clinic for seven months. Enquiry revealed that she had been well without any relapse and the post-coital burning was absent. She is still under observation and there has been no relapse to date.

Observation: This case taught me the efficacy of homeopathy in chronic recurrent diseases. The patient was well managed with antibiotics for about two decades, but her dependence on these kept increasing till she needed injectable antibiotics, which scared her. Homeopathy made her life comfortable and use of antibiotics was reduced.

PART FIVE

Experiments in the Field of Tuberculosis

Sixteen

Background

My interest in homeopathy had led me to teach medicine in a homeopathy medical college. The curriculum of the undergraduate course in homeopathy was surprisingly the same as that of modern medicine, except for pharmacology—the branch of medicine concerned with the uses, effects and modes of action of drugs. Students read the same books on all subjects except pharmacology. It was a revelation that the two systems differed only in the preparation of medicines and their principle of application in a disease.

In the last decade of the twentieth century (1995), I was preparing notes on tuberculosis (TB) to teach the final year students. A paragraph on epidemiology, hitherto gone unnoticed, struck my attention. It was about the risk of contracting infection and getting the disease. While contracting infection was by coming into contact with a person in overcrowded, indoor living with lack of ventilation and sunshine, developing pulmonary (lung) TB with a smear positive cough, depended on the healthy nasal mucosa and robust immune system of the recipient. Contracting infection and getting pulmonary TB were two different stages. One could contract infection by coming in close contact with a person suffering from pulmonary TB coughing out infected sputum, as in overcrowded indoor living with lack of ventilation and sunshine. Getting the disease, however, depended on the health of the recipient; if this person was malnourished and suffered from respiratory allergy, he/she would get pulmonary TB. But if the nasal passage was healthy and the immune system robust, the person may never suffer from the disease, but remained infected from latent infection. Such a person could get the disease any time, whenever the immunity was low for a prolonged length of time. Once infected, the person remained infected for many years, maybe all his/her life; but may never contract the disease. It was an interesting revelation from a homeopathy point of view, which is supposed to act on the immune system, making it robust, while antibiotics in modern medicine acted on the bacteria by killing/stopping the multiplication. It aroused my interest in the disease and I decided to go through the available literature.

The history of TB can be traced to ancient times when it was known as consumption/phthisis. The term 'Tuberculosis' was coined much later in 1834 by Johann Schonlein. It was found 9,000 years ago in the remains of a mother and child buried together in Atlit Yam, a city now under the Mediterranean Sea. The earliest written mentions of India were 3,300 years ago, and of China 2,300 years ago. Hippocrates identified phthisis as the most widespread disease which was always fatal around 460 BC, and with Galen, the Greek physician, formed the hygienic and dietetic regimen for its treatment.

TB caused immense public concern in the nineteenth and early twentieth centuries and was declared as an endemic disease of the urban poor. During this time, it killed one out of every seven people living in the United States and Europe. In 1815 England, one in four deaths were due to consumption. By 1880, TB was established as a contagious disease, hence notifiable. Dr Robert Koch, the German scientist who identified the TB bacterium, wrote *'one-seventh of all human beings die of tuberculosis, and if one considers only the productive middle-age groups, tuberculosis carries away one-third and often more of these'*. By 1918, one in six deaths in France were still caused by TB.

In this pre-chemotherapy era, when no anti-TB drugs were available, the emphasis was laid on early diagnosis and prevention of the disease. This was the era of adopting general hygienic measures, good nutrition and sanatoriums for treatment, with the first sanatorium opening in Poland in 1859. Homeopathic literature of this period abounds with stories of curing TB with homeopathy. Baron von Bonninghausen in 1827 was cured of purulent TB by A. Weihe (Doctor of Medicine [MD]) with the homeopathic medicine *Pulsatilla*, with advice on hygienic measures. Dr Hampel (1859) in his *Materia Medica* pointed out '*arsenic* excites in the respiratory organs, a process similar to phthisis' and used it in many cases. Taking the lead from Hampel, Dr Herbert Nankivell used *Ars.iod (3x)* in phthisis. British homeopath Richard Hughes in his book, *The Principles and Practice of Homeopathy* in 1878, advocated the use of different medicines for various stages of the disease along with fresh air, plenty of exercise, cod liver oil and chalybeate food (easily assimilable food). *Ars-i.* had become a standard medicine for phthisis in British homeopathic practice. Robert Koch in 1890 produced *Tuberculin*. The discovery of *Tuberculin* raised high hopes in patients but it failed due to overdosage. By about the end of 1890–92, Dr Burnett produced a brochure entitled 'Five years experience in the cure of consumption by its own virus', illustrated by 54 cases.

The bacillus causing TB, *Mycobacterium tuberculosis*, was described on 24 March 1882 by Robert Koch for which he received the Nobel Prize in physiology in 1905. This day of March is celebrated as World TB Day every year. The discovery of *Streptomycin* for the treatment of TB in 1944 was an important step in the history of medicine. For some time, it appeared that TB had been won over, but this euphoria lasted for a short time. Drug-resistance became a cause for concern in the management and control of the disease. This was countered by formulating various multiple drug regimes, Category I, II and III of four drugs followed by use of second-generation antibiotics and six to seven drugs at a time. There was increased focus on improved surveillance and diagnostic techniques to facilitate early detection of the disease and compliance of the drug regimen. The reliance on the efficacy of antibiotics was high and it was felt that prolonged regular use would lead to total eradication of the bacteria. But drug-resistance has continued to rise and has reached alarming proportions.

The forty-fourth World Health Assembly (WHA) in 1991 recognized the growing importance of TB and declared TB a public health emergency. In 1997, WHO formulated the Directly Observed Treatment Short Course (DOTS) strategy. The cure rates among patients harbouring multidrug-resistant isolates ranged from 6 to 59 per cent.

The Indian National Tuberculosis Control Programme (NTCP) was launched in 1962 and the revised (RNTCP) in 1993 for the prevention and control of the disease.

FIGURE 1: Far advanced X-ray changes in case no. 184 showing Grade +5 improvement

A

Before treatment

Far advanced changes

- Multiple cavities in right upper zone and mid zone, size more than 4 cm in diameter
- Dense and confluent shadow seen in lower half of right lung
- Infiltration present in the left lung
- Presence of bilateral hilar enlargement

B

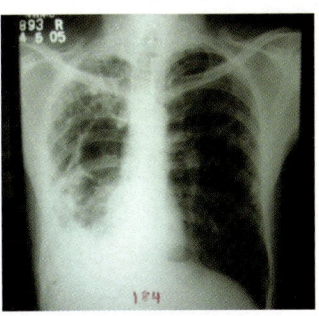

After 1 year of treatment

- Size of cavity reduced
- Healing with fibrosis
- Dense infiltrate of right side getting cleared
- Left side infiltration getting cleared

C

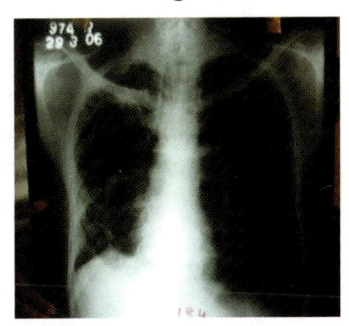

After 1 year six months of treatment

- Complete resolution of cavity and infiltration in right lung with minimum fibrosis
- Absence of infiltration in left lung with compensatory hypertrophy

FIGURE 2: Far advanced changes in case no. 172 showing -4 deterioration

A

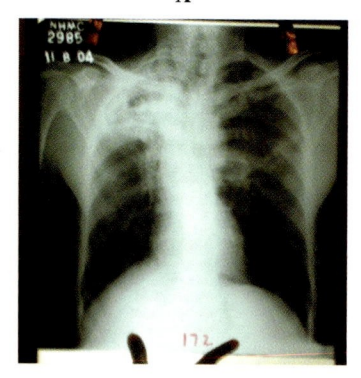

Before treatment

- Confluent cavities with dense shadow in right upper lobe with infiltration in mid zone
- Infiltration in left upper and mid zone and bilateral hilar nodes enlargement

B

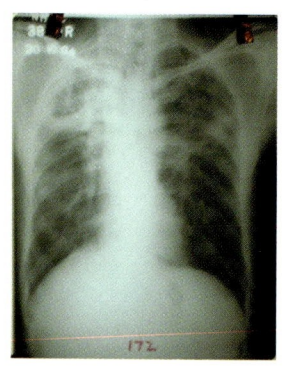

After two months of treatment

- Increase in size of all lesions
- Confluent cavities with dense shadow in right upper lobe with infiltration in mid zone
- Infiltration in left upper and mid zone and bilateral hilar nodes enlargement

C

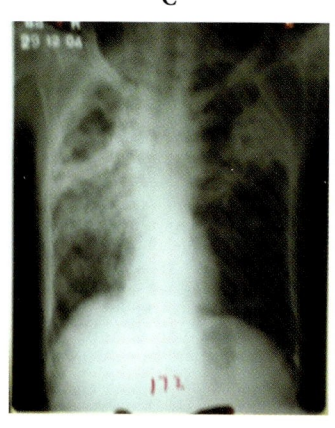

After four months of treatment

- Increase in size of the cavities and infiltration seen on right side
- Increased area of infiltration with cavity on left side

FIGURE 3

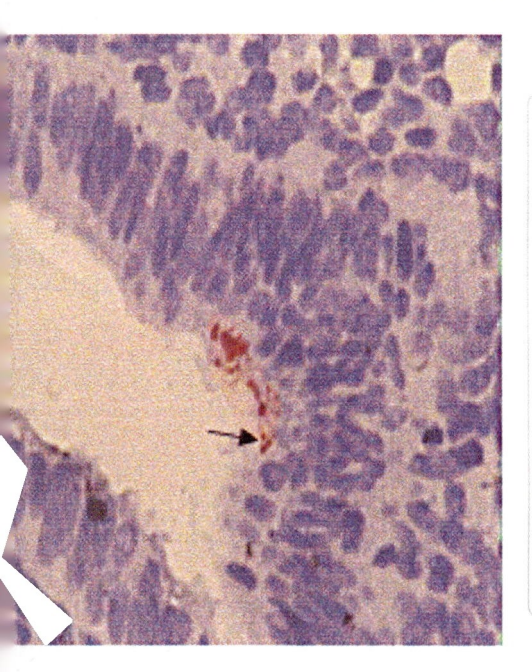

FIGURE 4

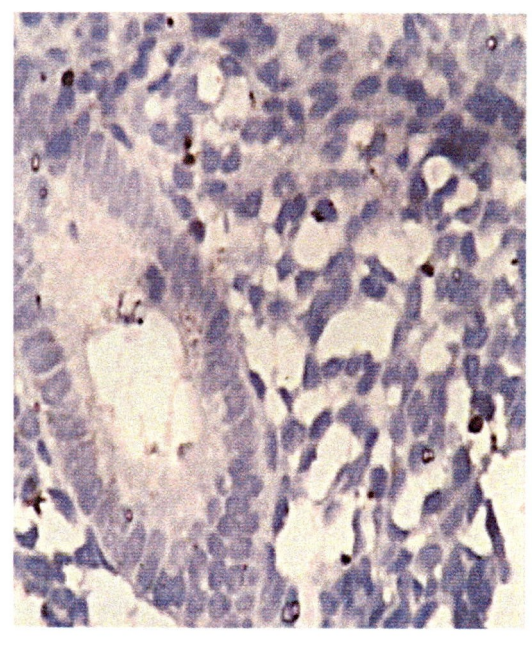

FIGURE 5

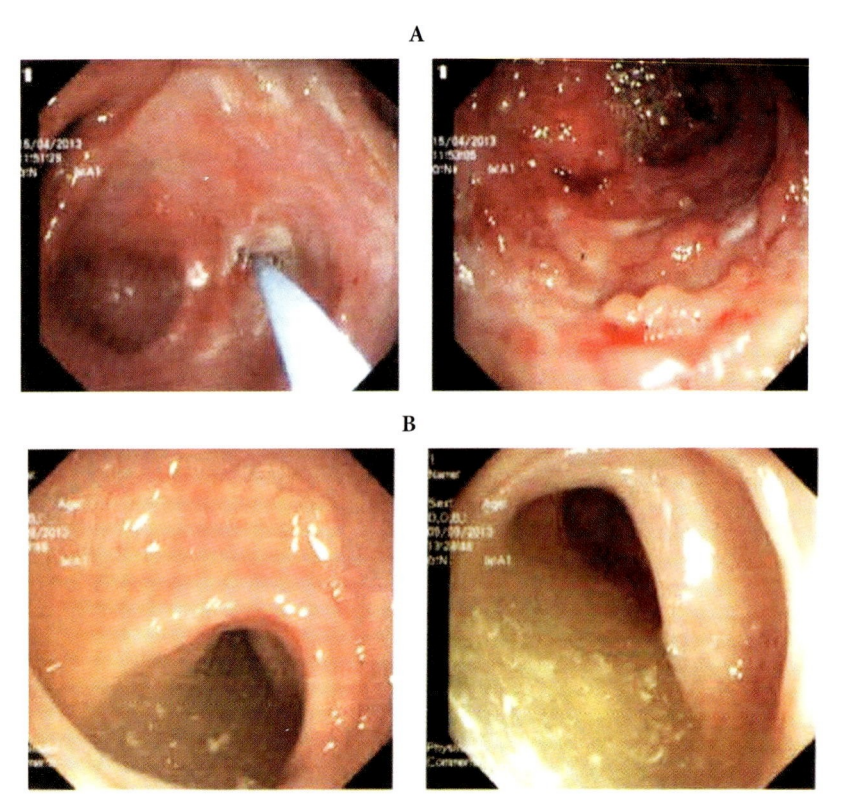

A e Colonoscopy (15/04/13) showed nodular lesion in ascending colon, ulceration and nodular lesions involving the ileo caecal valve, possible ileo caecal Koch's; B e Colonoscopy (09/09/13) showed. Compared to previous findings there is complete healing of ulcers with contracted caecum.

FIGURE 6

Chest radiographs of case 3. A e 01/04/2015 shows prominent hilar with fibrotic lesions in right lung. B e 01/07/2015 hilar less prominent. C e 06/01/2016 hilar normal and fibrotic lesions much reduced.

FIGURE 7

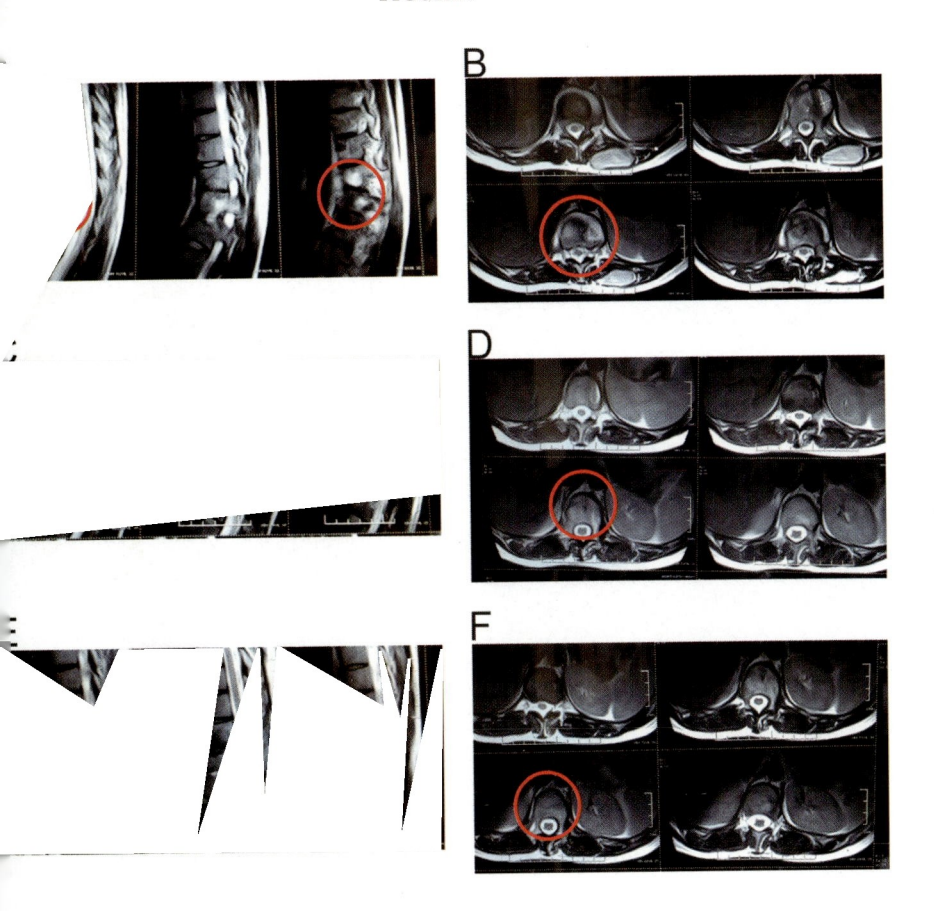

Figure 6 MRI reports of case 1. 07/09/2014 MRI dorsal spine A e features suggestive of tubercular spine with destructive pathology involving D8 to L1 vertebral bodies; B e pre/paravertebral and left-sided paraspinal muscular collection of fluid; 13/06/2015 C e partial resolution of the pathology with healing at D8 to L1 vertebral bodies and persisting infective lesion at D10, D11, D12 level; D e minimal pre-vertebral collection of fluid; 07/11/2015 E e near complete resolution of the pathology with healing at D8 to D11 vertebral bodies with persisting discitis of D12eL1 level; F e no evidence of collection of fluid seen.

FIGURE 8

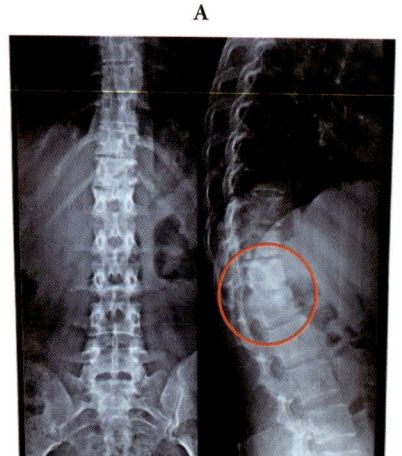

A   B

X-ray Spine 8A shows fracture of vertebra 8B shows no bony lesion

FIGURE 9

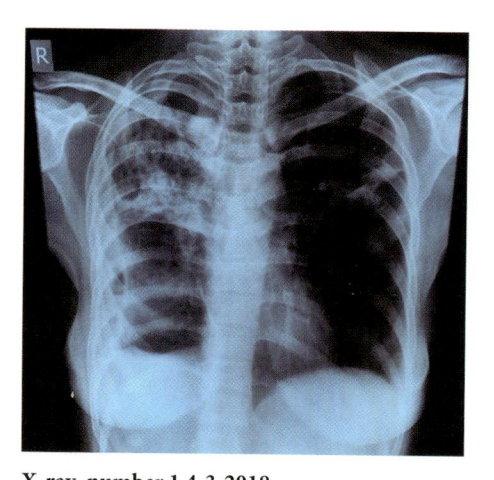

X-ray number 1 4-3-2018

- Both lungs are hyperinflated
- Right apical pleura thickened
- Large infiltrate is seen in the right upper lobe with central cavitation
- Right hilum is enlarged ? nodes
- Loculated and free pleural effusion along right chest wall
- Focal infiltration also seen in left upper lobe

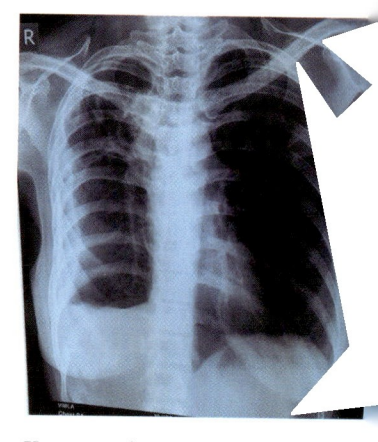

X-ray number 5 7-5-2019

- Thick-walled cavity in right upper lobe is thin-walled with no surrounding infiltrate
- Right-sided pleural effusion/ thickening is status quo
- Left lung is clear

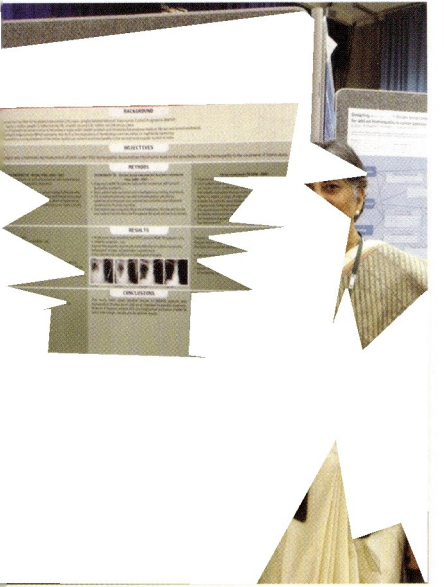

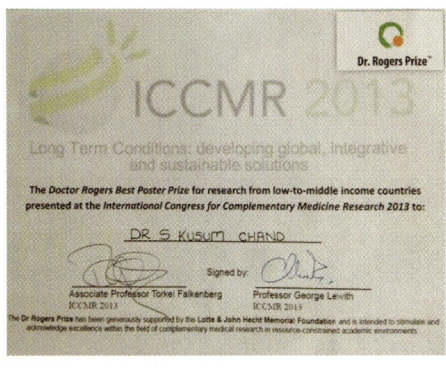

Doctor Rogers' Prize for the Best Poster for Research

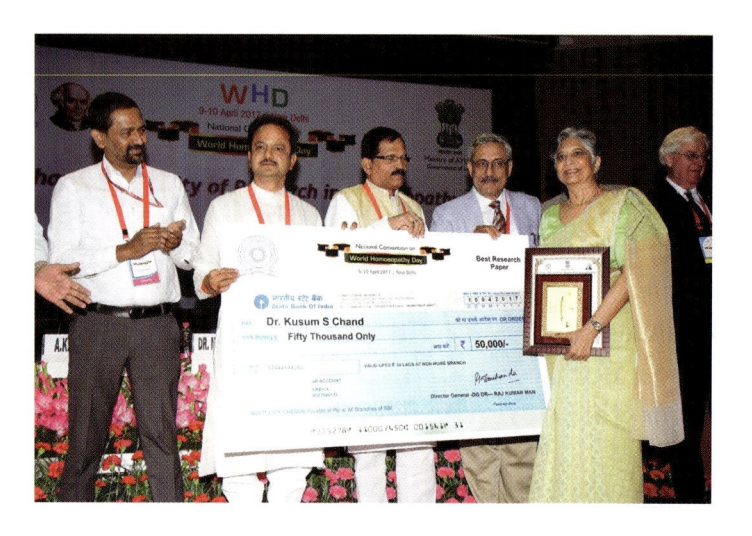

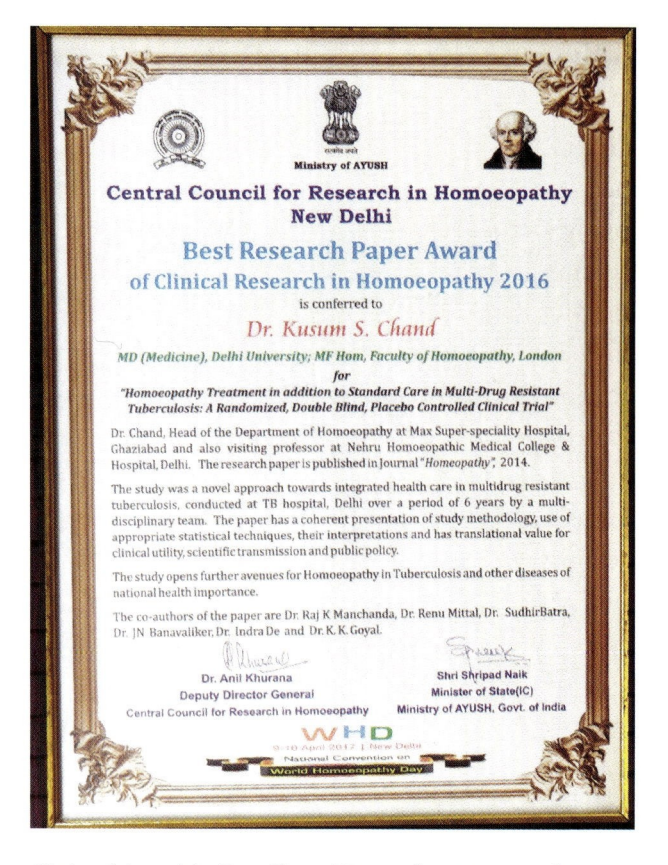

National Award for Best Clinical Research in Homeopathy, 2017

Patients were divided into three categories and antitubercular treatment (ATT) consisted of regimes of multiple antibiotics. 'Category I (Cat I) consists of thrice weekly doses of: *Isoniazid (INH), Rifampicin (R), Ethambutol (ETH), Pyrazinamide (PYZ)* for two months, then *INH and R* for four months. It is given to new smear-positive, seriously ill smear-negative and seriously ill extra pulmonary cases. Category II (Cat II) consists of thrice weekly doses of: *INH, R, ETH, PYZ, Streptomycin (STR)* for two months, then *INH, R, ETH, PYZ* for one month, then *INH, R, ETH* for five months. It is given to smear-positive, relapse, failed and default cases. Category III (CAT III) consists of thrice weekly doses of: *INH, R, PYZ* for two months, then *INH, R* for four months. It is given to non-seriously ill, smear-negative and extra pulmonary cases. DOTS Course strategy has been adopted to reduce default rate and increase the compliance of a patient. ATT is administered in front of a physician or a health worker.'

The *Mycobacterium* causing TB has successfully countered all efforts of mankind in controlling its pathogenicity and eradicating the disease. It has done so by having a cell wall that can resist the action of antibiotics and has evolved multiple strategies to modulate innate immune responses and prevent optimal activation of the adaptive immunity of the host so as to lie dormant inside the macrophage without replication for years. Bacteria transmitted from a person suffering from pulmonary TB in the sputum are likely to be metabolically active. They have the capacity to activate the dormant bacteria of the recipient host.

Study of the patho-physiology of TB revealed that only 10 per cent of the bacteria reached the pulmonary alveoli after exposure to infection, the balance 90 per cent were thrown out by the action of healthy mucosa lining the upper respiratory tract. In the alveoli, bacteria were ingested by the non-specifically activated macrophages. The degree of bactericidal activity of macrophages was dependent on innate non-specific immune resistance to infection. Once infected (latent TB), a person could develop TB at any time and only 10 per cent of infected persons developed the active disease (attack rate was 1 in 1000). This meant that the host's response to infection is quite efficacious in containing the pathogen but inefficacious in eradicating it. The progression of latent TB to active disease was directly related to a patient's degree of immune-suppression and clusters of differentiation (CD4) + cell count. Various physical or emotional stresses could trigger progression of infection to disease due to weakening of the immune system. The higher incidence of TB observed in chronic diseases—diabetes, alcoholic liver disease, HIV co-infection, the use of steroids or other immune-suppressive drugs, increasing use of biological drugs, such as tumour necrosis factor-α (TNF-α)/Interleukin (IL)-12/IL-23 blockers for the treatment of inflammatory diseases like rheumatoid arthritis, Crohn's disease, and psoriasis—is deemed to be due to perturbations of the immune system.

It is evident from the above study of pathology that the state of immunity of a person has an important role in progression of infection to disease. Allopathic medicine was focused on the immediate external cause: the microbe; while immunity was taken for granted, which waxed and waned with the physical and mental state of a person. Homeopathic literature had mentions of the usefulness of homeopathy in the treatment of TB. The thought of a two-pronged approach: target the microbe and improve the immunity simultaneously was an exciting dream for me.

Seventeen

The Project:
Role of Homeopathy In Tuberculosis

Soon an opportunity came my way to work in the field of tuberculosis (TB). An article was published in 1998 in the journal *Homeopathy*, indicating the usefulness of the addition of homeopathy in the treatment of pulmonary TB. In 1999, a project to study the role of homeopathy in the treatment of TB was initiated by the Government of Delhi, India, in collaboration with a specialized TB hospital. Category II patients were to be studied from the homeopathic perspective by a team of seven experts: five senior research officers and two specialists. I was one of the specialists. After noting the symptoms and understanding the constitution of the patient, a suitable homeopathic medicine was selected, following discussion among team members. The presence of at least one specialist was mandatory. The selected medicine was given as an add-on treatment to the ongoing allopathic ATT. Follow-up was every two weeks.

The project started at the Nehru Homeopathic Medical College (NHMC), Defence Colony, New Delhi. While the patient had to take the allopathic treatment from various DOT centres across the city, they needed to come to Nehru Medical College for their homeopathic treatment. This was inconvenient in the sense that the two clinics were at two different places, quite far from each other. A patient had to take two days' leave and also spend on transport to go to two clinics. Patients were from the lower income group, with many being daily wage-earners. This resulted in low attendance by the end of the year. Hence, a second clinic was opened at the TB Hospital at Nehru Nagar. This was better as the patient got both treatments at the same place. The NHMC clinic continued to be where mostly tubercular lymphadenopathy patients and those referred from adjacent DOTS clinics were treated.

I was excited, yet sceptical, of the efficacy of homeopathy in a disease where powerful specific antibiotics were failing. One morning, I was called by the project manager to see a patient of diarrhoea. The latter was a case of intestinal TB, recently operated on. In the operation a part of the intestines had been removed. Her frequent stools with fever had not responded to allopathic treatment, hence she was referred by the TB specialist associated with the project. I was sceptical of the effectiveness of homeopathy in such a case, yet prescribed medicine for one week according to her symptoms. To my pleasant surprise, the patient reported marked improvement in the frequency of stools and fever. Thus began my journey in the management of TB.

In three years, from 2000 to 2003, in the first phase of the project, 142 CAT II failure patients suffering from pulmonary TB were studied. Along with them, about fifty cases of tubercular lymphadenitis were treated, who were either close family relations of the above patients or cases referred from the adjacent DOTS clinic. After success in the first phase, an exploratory randomized, double-blind, parallel group placebo-controlled study was conducted from June 2003 to March 2008.

This was a period of deep thinking, logical analysis and experimentation for me.

Eighteen

Outcome of the Project

First phase

The object was to study the effect of the addition of homeopathic medicine to the standard treatment protocol of allopathic medicine. These patients were referred from TB chest clinics. In three years, 142 patients (Category II failure) on the second course of ATT were studied. There was regular follow-up of up to one year for 94 patients.

Add-on homeopathy was found to be effective in drug-intolerant patients. There was symptomatic improvement and reduction in frequency of acute episodes in other patients.

The twelve most often used medicines were shortlisted: *Arsenic album (Ars.) 30c, Bryonia (Bry.) 30c, 200c, Calcarea carbonica (Calc.) 30c, Ipecacuanha (Ip.) 30c, Lycopodium (Lyc.) 30, Natrum muriaticum (Nat-m.) 30, Nux vomica (Nux-v.) 30, Phosphorus (Phos.) 30c, 200c, Pulsatilla nigricans (Puls.) 30c, Sepia (Sep.) 30c, 200c, Sulphur (Sulph.) 30c* and *Tuberculinum bovinum (Tub.) 200c*. It was felt that homeopathy could be useful in the management of TB and approval for a double-blind randomized placebo-controlled trial was sought from the Scientific Advisory Committee (SAC) and the Institutional Ethical Committee.

Final Randomized Controlled Trial (RCT)

An exploratory randomized, double-blind, parallel group, placebo-controlled study was conducted from June 2003 to March 2008. The location was a specialized DOTS centre, where diagnosed Multidrug Resistant (MDR) TB patients were treated with second generation (reserve line) antibiotics. This was the Standard Regimen (SR) as per RNTCP guidelines. A homeopathy centre was created within the same premises.

Patients were diagnosed as MDR TB on the basis of a Drug Sensitivity Test (DST). Patients from all age groups, with varying duration of illness and current culture status were enrolled in the study. Both culture positive (new) (n = 81), and culture negative, but still symptomatic (being treated with the SR) (n = 39) patients were referred by the TB chest specialist, Dr Jayant N. Banavaliker (JNB) to the homeopathic centre. Further assessment of eligibility was conducted by the homeopathic doctors. Pregnant women and patients with concomitant diseases such as HIV or malignancy were excluded. Patients were enrolled from June 2003 to April 2005.

Written prior informed consent was obtained from each participant/guardian.

A standardized patient case record form was used for recording the symptoms, details of previous ATT and investigations. All patients were given the SR with add-on homeopathic medicine.

Allopathic treatment SR comprised six drugs: *Kanamycin,*

Levofloxacin, Ethionamide, Pyrazinamide, Ethambutol and *Cycloserine* during six to nine months of the intensive phase, and four drugs: *Levofloxacin, Ethionamide, Ethambutol* and *Cycloserine* during eighteen months of the continuation phase. Patients were advised to take a nutritious diet and instructed about safe sputum disposal. The medicines were dispensed from an outpatient department under the RNTCP, after the patient had visited the homeopathy centre. This system proved to be helpful in minimizing dropouts and achieving targets.

Homeopathic intervention consisted of treatment with pre-defined fifteen medicines that were shortlisted during the initial trial phase. A medicine box, consisting of fifteen two-drachm glass vials, each labelled with the name of one of the medicines, was prepared. Homeopathic intervention was blinded, in the medicinal group (SR + H) the vial was filled with labelled medicine and in the placebo group (SR + P), it was filled with pills soaked in ethyl alcohol. Initially, fifty boxes were prepared, serially numbered and randomized by the project director. The allocation ratio between the two groups was kept as 1:1. After 100, 150 boxes were prepared in one go to eliminate bias. These boxes were kept in the pharmacy section.

Each patient was assigned one medicine box at the time of enrolment in the project. The enrolment number and the medicine box number were the same for a patient. The patient received medicine from the same box throughout the study period. I found this to be an effective and practical way. Blinding was done at the NHMC office by the project manager, who did not see the patients and the prescribers and pharmacist at the project unit had nothing to do with the blinding process. The patients received the intervention either as SR + individualized homeopathic medicine (SR + H) or SR + placebo (SR + P).

In all, 220 patients were enrolled.

The experiment was unblinded by Raj K. Manchanda (RKM) at the end of the study period (2008) after the blind assessment of all parameters. The clinical status was evaluated by Kusum Chand (KC, myself) and Sudhir Batra (SB) and chest X-rays (CXRs) by the team of Jayant N. Banavaliker (JNB) and Indra De (ID). Outcome measures used were sputum smear and culture conversion, radiological changes, haemoglobin (Hb), Erythrocytic Sedimentation Rate (ESR), weight gain and change in clinical symptoms. The patients were followed up every fifteen days for clinical assessment in terms of absence (0) or presence (1) of eight common symptoms—cough, pain in chest, haemoptysis, expectoration, lassitude, anorexia, dyspnoea and fever—to calculate symptom score. Weight in kilograms (kg) was recorded. Sputum smear and culture were assessed at three months' interval. The tests for Hb and ESR (Wintrobe's method) were conducted at the baseline and at the end. CXRs were evaluated at six-month intervals and grading of each CXR was done by two chest specialists, (JNB) and a senior clinical radiologist (ID), independently using the classification of the National Tuberculosis Association of USA.

The data was first analysed using the Glasgow Homoeopathic Hospital Outcome Scale (GHHOS) criteria, which was unable to bring out the difference between the two groups and the study was shelved. It was a complex study in a chronic disease where healing left scars on the lung tissue, leading to permanent structural changes on CXRs and continued symptoms like cough and breathlessness.

Prolonged use of drugs could lead to chronic nutritional deficiency. Though the disease was cured, some symptoms remained. Hence the difference would be qualitative rather than quantitative.

The two prescribers, SB, Renu Mittal (RM) and consultant KC strongly felt the difference; analysis of CXRs by JNB also showed substantial improvement in the SR + H group. ID had commented that CXRs of some patients showed appearance of new lesions, which healed without fibrosis; these CXRs belonged to the SR + H group.

Hence the data of 120 patients was reanalysed by KC, SB and RM with the enrolment numbers from 101 to 220. The first 100 patients from 1 to 100 were not considered as there was irregularity in case taking and late prescribing of indicated medicine due to delay in setting up and proper functioning of the homeopathy centre.

The data of 120 patients was analysed by the Statistical Package for Social Sciences (SPSS 20.0) in two ways: (i) intention to treat (ITT) approach with last observation carried forward (LOCF) to impute 18.3 per cent of missing data (ii) per protocol (PP) for patients with minimum two culture reports and two CXRs. Thirteen patients did not have two culture reports and nine patients did not have two CXRs at the completion of the study; thus, the PP analysis involved only 98 patients, 49 in each group. Analysis of culture positive and culture negative patients was done as subgroups.

Computing the findings of CXRs was a difficult task. If viewed alone, every CXR showed far advanced changes at the beginning of the study and remained so till the end; yet the comparison of CXRs of a patient, at the beginning and end of the study, revealed varying differences from better to worse. After much thought and approval of chest specialists, JNB and ID, a Radiological Assessment Tool (RAT) was developed. Radiological change was graded from +5 to -5, no change was 0, seen in twenty-one patients; maximum improvement in three (Figure 1, see p. 1 of insert) and maximum deterioration in one (Figure 2, see p. 2 of insert).

The culture positive and negative patients were also analysed as separate subgroups using the assessment criteria of RNTCP.

The culture negative patients were assessed for change in clinical symptoms and for the recurrence rate (culture conversion from negative to positive).*

This was/is the first clinical study based on the RCT model to evaluate the efficacy of add-on homeopathy to the standard conventional treatment regimen followed in the treatment of MDR TB. All the patients were diagnosed cases of MDR TB, based on sputum culture positivity and DST results. They had far advanced pulmonary lesions, were nutritionally compromised with drug effects from prolonged use of antibiotics.

The patients were allotted batch numbers randomly without consideration of age, sex and severity of disease, yet baseline statistics revealed that the groups were comparable in term of assessment variables.

Sputum smear conversion was marginally lower (1.7 per cent), whereas culture conversion was 11.4 per cent more

---

*The detailed analysis can be accessed in an original article published in the journal *Homeopathy*. Chand, K.S., Manchanda, R.K., Mittal, R., Batra, S., Banavaliker, J.N., De, I. 'Homeopathic treatment in addition to standard care in multi drug resistant pulmonary tuberculosis: A randomized, double blind, placebo-controlled clinical trial', *Homeopathy*, 2014, 103: 97–107.

and time taken for culture conversion was shorter with add-on homeopathy. However results were not statistically significant, hence this intervention appeared to have no substantial effect on sputum conversion.

Statistically highly significant ($p = 0.0005$) improvement in CXRs was an important finding of this study, suggestive of a T helper-1 (Th1) type of response, which results in less inflammation, no immunopathology (necrosis) and fibrosis, while inflammation and tissue remodelling with pathologic fibrosis are common consequences of Th2 responses in the lung and other organs. It is said that much of the immune response to *Mycobacterium tuberculosis* is involved in immunopathology, not immunity.

There had been statistically significant improvement in weight ($p = 0.026$) and haemoglobin ($p = 0.017$) and reduction in ESR ($p = 0.025$) in the homeopathy group, which are parameters of acute disease process. The symptom score had been almost the same in both groups, indicating the persistence of symptoms due to the chronic sequel of the disease. Highest improvement was observed in the subgroup analysis of culture positive patients where homeopathic intervention was started early along with the standard regimen.

Experiments with tubercular lymphadenopathy

The NHMC centre also had patients suffering from tubercular lymphadenopathy coming in for treatment. Since this form of TB is not contagious, it was not ethically mandatory to put them on allopathic ATT. One could treat them with only homeopathy.

These cases were separate from the ongoing project.

We had seen fifty patients. The protocol was to include any patient who had lymph nodes larger than 1.5 cm^2 anywhere in the body. Such a patient was investigated for haemoglobin, TLC and DLC, ESR, radiological assessment of the chest and FNAC of the enlarged lymph node either before or within fifteen days of start of treatment. Patient was reviewed every fortnight. Treatment was homeopathy for all the complaints. If the patient was on allopathic ATT, he/she was allowed to continue the treatment.

The aim was to achieve a cure of symptoms, as well as reduction in size of lymph nodes in the shortest time, without any aggravation. The protocol of the classical method of one medicine at a time was modified according to our experiences in the following steps:

The first step was to treat the cases with homeopathy alone, single indicated remedy, repeated only when there was no improvement at any level. This method showed partial improvement. The lymph nodes regressed only partially. As the general symptoms showed improvement and the lymph nodes stopped regressing in size, the patients stopped attending the clinic.

The second step was to give the constitutional medicine at regular intervals, even if there was improvement in symptoms.

The third step was to give *Tuberculinum* in 200c to a patient of active TB at infrequent intervals, whenever the improvement with constitutional medicine stopped.

The fourth step was to treat the acute symptoms—fever, cold, cough, bowel disturbances and so on—with indicated homeopathic remedies along with constitutional remedy.

The fifth step was the regular use of indicated constitutional remedy and nosode *Tuberculinum* along with a general stimulant *Sil. 6D*. Constitutional remedy was repeated at weekly or even lesser intervals, and *Tub. 200c* at weekly and *Tub. 1M* at fortnightly intervals; *Sil. 6D* was given daily.

The assessment of the response and duration of treatment was guided by mainly the reduction in size and number of lymph nodes, along with an absence of symptoms and gain in weight.

The treatment stopped when the lymph nodes became soft and size reduced to less than one cm.[2.]

Results: Fifty patients were registered, there was a regular follow-up of forty-seven patients.

In twelve patients the FNAC report was invalid—either it could not be performed or it was performed much later after the start of treatment.

Five patients were lost at the first step of treatment protocol. As the general symptoms improved and lymph nodes stopped regressing, patients stopped attending the clinic.

Five case histories were lost during transfer of the clinic.

Complete recovery of constitutional symptoms was observed in all these cases. Lymph nodes became impalpable in eleven cases and reduced by 75 per cent in the remaining fourteen cases.

Retrospective study of fifty cases of tubercular lymphadenitis (TBLN) revealed that in twenty-five cases, the records were complete according to protocol: all the investigations, particularly the FNAC, were done either before or within fifteen days of starting the treatment.

Follow-up of all cases till the end stage was available, in a few, a longer follow-up was also present.

The summary of these cases of TBLN giving details of the onset and duration of disease, investigations, selection of remedies from the individualized repertory graph (RG), duration and outcome of treatment is given below.

The cases have been placed in chronological order to highlight the evolution of the treatment regimen.

Based on this analysis, a paper by Chand, S.K., Manchanda, R.K., Batra, S., Mittal, R. titled, 'Homeopathy in the Treatment of Tubercular Lymphadenitis—An Indian Experience', was published in the journal *Homeopathy*. *Homeopathy*, 2011, 100 (3): 157–67.

Nineteen

Idea of Formation of a Homeopathic Regime

We began with the treatment protocol: that after detailed history and panel discussions, a suitable medicine would be selected, which was to be dispensed as a single dose, followed by the placebo. If the patient said that his/her symptoms were improving on the follow-up visit after two weeks, only the placebo was prescribed on the principle 'repeat the dose, only after the effect of the previous medicine is over'. The medicinal dose was repeated only when the improvement became static and it was reselected if there was no change in symptoms. If the patient had an acute episode of a seasonal disease, it was not treated on the principle that the old symptoms were coming back and a medicinal dose would take care of it, but the patient was troubled and sought treatment from a general physician.

This set me thinking that for the treatment of his/her disease, the patient was already visiting two centres, a DOTS centre for TB drugs and another for general symptoms. He/she would come for homeopathy, only if it offered a comprehensive treatment plan, with perceptible advantage.

Homeopathy literature was full of instances where the allopathic system had failed and homeopathy had led to a complete cure. I felt if incurable cases could be treated, then TB could also be amenable to homeopathy. There were treatment protocols for every disease in allopathy, so why not in homeopathy?

Single dose: The practice of a single dose in homeopathy put questions in my mind. If the treatment of TB was so simple, then we would not have an epidemic of TB cases. Also, we were attributing all the beneficial effects to a single dose of homeopathic medicine, while the patient was also on a full regime of allopathic ATT.

Repetition of dose: The duration of action of the medicine was another question mark. We were going by what was written in books, which were at best general statements not specific to the disease or a patient. I started interrogating patients about their reaction to the medicinal dose. Their feedback was that the improvement lasted from one to three/four days, then became static at the new level. So, on their subsequent visit to the clinic, the statement 'I am better' meant that they were better than the first visit, but it did not mean that the effect of the dose was continuing. To me the patient needed another dose. Under the chapter 'Calcarea Carbonica' in Kent's *Materia Medica* (p. 323), it is mentioned: 'Here is another thing I have seen: even when there were no symptoms left, and after waiting a considerable time and there were no symptoms, I have seen another dose of the same medicine that was given on the last symptoms, gave the patient a great lift, and pathological conditions commence to go away.' This boosted my conviction for a repetition of the dose, even when symptoms were improving, but the pathology continued.

Pulmonary TB treated with only homeopathy: Experiment 1

The director of the project admitted a poor patient from the street. He had a cough with bloody sputum and moderate fever. The investigations revealed him to be suffering from pulmonary TB with pleural effusion. He was isolated in one room and treatment started with Lyc. 30c, *three doses in a day followed by* Fer-p. 6D *three times a day. A dose of* Lyc. 200c *was given after three days,* Fer-p. 6D *continued as before. There was no change in fever or the patient's general condition. My advice of a daily dose of* Lyc. 200c *and* Fer-p. 6D *three times a day met with resistance, but was nullified by the director. The fever started receding after a week; his cough was treated successfully with* Kali-c. 30c *and* Grindalia *mother tincture. Within two months, the patient began gaining in weight; cough and sputum were scanty; pleural effusion became less.*

This case further strengthened my conviction of repeating the dose.

Use of certain medicines

Homeopathic literature had conflicting views on the use of certain medicines in the treatment of this disease. Hence, in the beginning, the Scientific Advisory Committee (SAC) had cautioned against the use of *Phosphorus, Silicea, Sulphur* and *Tuberculinum*. Symptom-wise, these were indicated, but some had experienced adverse effects, hence the caution against their use. After much thought, I felt that it was not the fault of the medicine but of its potency and the manner of its use. I felt *Phosphorus* and *Sulphur* could be useful in medium potency in infrequent doses.

Pulmonary TB treated with only homeopathy: Experiment 2

By the end of 2000, word had spread about our project. A man came seeking for help in homeopathy for his young daughter. She was suffering from pulmonary TB, and was being treated with allopathic ATT. Lately, she had become intolerant of the drugs and had constant nausea, vomiting and fever, to the extent that ATT had to be withdrawn. The homeopathic medicine was Phos., *but how to dispense it was a dilemma. Her condition demanded frequent doses, hence it was given in millesimal (LM) potency (useful in a sensitive patient, as it could be given more frequently without fear of aggravation) to avoid aggravation. She responded well and within ten days was without fever and eating well. We requested the father to continue with homeopathy but he was of the opinion that only one system of medicine should be followed at a time and preferred allopathic medicine.*

Study of *Silicea* gave me the idea that it could be used both as a constitutional medicine (based on symptom similarity) and as a non-specific general stimulant of phagocytic (killing) activity of leucocytes giving protection against the pus-producing bacteria. The bacteria could be *Staphylococcus, Streptococcus* or *Tubercular bacillus*. For the latter action, decimal potency was recommended. This appealed to me and was tried in cases of tubercular adenitis, giving the constitutional medicine as one dose a week, followed by six days of *Silicea 6x*. This way, some medicinal anti-tubercular activity was ensured every day.

I was excited and keen to experiment with the use of *Tuberculinum* in the treatment of active disease. If Burnett in the nineteenth century could cure TB, it certainly was worth validating it now. Most of the senior homeopaths were sceptical of its use in the active disease except for Dr Bansi Dhar, who felt that it could be useful in the treatment of active disease like Burnett had proved.

Twenty

Experiences In a Hospital Setting

This project convinced me that homeopathy could be usefully employed in the management of TB. In 2008, I joined the department of Complementary and Alternate Medicine (CAM) in a multispeciality tertiary care hospital as the head of the homeopathy department. In my clinical practice of general medicine without hospital attachment, I saw patients in the earlier stages of disease. Though the results with homeopathy were satisfying and I had a good practice, yet the idea of working in a hospital setting was exciting. The thought was to get the opportunity to see patients with difficult multimorbidities and experiment with integrating homeopathy with mainstream allopathy.

The yearly 2008 WHO report 'Stop TB Strategy' on World TB Day was disheartening. The microbe *Mycobacterium tuberculosis* remained untamed. All the strategies and antibiotics could not control the havoc caused by it in public healthcare. It said that: 'MDR-TB continues to threaten the progress made in controlling the disease. The emergence of extensively drug-resistant TB (XDR-TB), defined as MDR-TB, that is resistant as well to any one of the fluoroquinolones and to at least one of three injectable second-line drugs (amikacin, capreomycin or kanamycin), has heightened this threat. XDR-TB has been identified in all regions of the world since 2006. Treatment outcomes are significantly worse in XDR-TB patients than in MDR-TB patients. Outbreaks of XDR-TB in populations with high prevalence of HIV have caused alarmingly high mortality rates. The emergence of XDR-TB is a new threat to global public health'. TB declared as global epidemic?

My experiences of treating drug-intolerant, drug-resistant TB cases, along with mainstream medicine, have been revealing and thought-provoking. The integration is easy and cost-effective. If followed, it can have a significant impact on the control of the disease. Following are some case histories. A few have been published in peer-reviewed journals.

Homeopathy in drug intolerance

Infertility with genital TB

My colleague from the gastroenterology department called me one day in 2010 to find out whether homeopathy had something for the treatment of TB. On being informed of my experience in TB, he referred the case of a twenty-two-year-old woman who had come to the infertility clinic with a complaint of irregular menses and primary infertility. An endometrial biopsy (Figure 3, see p. 3 of insert) on 8 May 2010 showed the presence of *Mycobacterium tuberculosis*, seen as clusters of tiny fuchsia pink rods. She was put on conventional ATT with a combination of four antibiotics: Isoniazid, Rifampicin, Ethambutol and Pyrazinamide (*Akt4*). Four weeks later, she suffered from severe dysmenorrhoea (painful menses), associated with anorexia and vomiting.

Her liver enzymes were raised, indicating drug-induced hepatitis. *Akt4* was replaced with different ATT drugs: Injectable *Streptomycin* and *Mycobutol,* along with liver drugs, Udiliv and Analiv. After ten days, when the level of raised liver enzymes fell down, two more ATT drugs *Risorine* and *Oflox,* were added. The patient complained of irritation in the eyes, difficulty in vision and acidity after three weeks of this treatment but the same treatment was continued for another three weeks, taking these symptoms as minor irritants in the face of a serious disease. The liver enzymes were again elevated after eleven weeks of this treatment, along with severe pain in the upper abdomen. *Risorine* was withdrawn immediately and all other drugs had to be stopped after a week due to severe eye symptoms.

A homeopathic view was asked for at this point.

The homeopathic prescription was based on the history of delayed and prolonged menses since menarche at the age of thirteen years; menses every three months, lasting for one and a half months; profuse leucorrhoea staining the line; aversion to coitus which was associated with burning during the act; throbbing headache made worse by talking; disturbed sleep from worry due to inability to conceive. Patient had a pale, sallow complexion, was sad and wept while talking and on her own admission, was short-tempered. Three medicines came out strongly: *Nat-m.* for mental symptoms, *Sep.* for location of the disease in the uterus, *Phos.* for drug-induced acute hepatitis and no appetite. I decided to address the disease at all the levels simultaneously; *Nat-m.* was given twice a week, *Sep.* five days a week, *Phos.* twice a day all days of the week along with disease-specific *Tub.* once a week. Prescription was for two weeks, but those two weeks were very long two weeks. Every day I was accosted either in the corridors of the hospital or on telephone to affirm the efficacy of homeopathy in such a serious disease as TB. By the end, I started doubting the efficacy myself. Came the fifteenth day and also the patient. I and my associate, Dr Priya Kapoor, looked at her and our eyes popped out. The pale sallow complexion had acquired a pinkish hue and instead of a sad weepy expression, there was a small smile. My breaking the rule of one medicine at a time was well rewarded. I did not care as long as it benefited the patient. Symptom-wise, the headache was 60 per cent less, leucorrhoea 20 per cent less and burning during coitus better by 50 per cent. Sleep was sound. Since there was improvement without any change in symptoms, the treatment was repeated for another two weeks. On her third visit, the liver enzymes had progressively reduced. The menstrual cycle was painless with good flow. She was getting hormonal treatment from an infertility clinic. Leucorrhoea had increased but was non-offensive and not staining. Burning during coitus and aversion to coitus was as before which she herself admitted in her husband's presence. As her symptoms and liver enzymes had markedly improved, frequency of *Phos.* was reduced to three doses a week and since the uterine symptoms were same, the dose of *Sep.* was increased to twice a day. Rest of the medicines remained the same.

When she came after a month, there was a marked improvement in her uterine symptoms. In between this period, during her visit to the infertility clinic, the gynaecologist at the clinic, on finding her to be looking bright and healthy, had advised a repeat of endometrial biopsy and liver function tests. All the liver function tests were normal and the fuchsia pink tiny rods were absent from the biopsy on 5 October 2010 (Figure 4, see p. 3 of insert). This was an unbelievable result: two months of homeopathy and the patient was cured of TB. Treatment continued for the next two months though *Phos.* was stopped as liver function tests were normal and appetite was good. After two months, a pelvic scan was performed to diagnose the cause of pain in the lower abdomen, which showed signs of pelvic inflammation. This was treated with *Thuj.* and *Bry.* In January, an Intra Uterine Insemination (IUI) procedure was performed and in February, the pregnancy test came positive.

Observation: This case was treated with only homeopathy, except for menstrual-regulating hormones, after allopathic drugs proved ineffective. Drug-induced hepatitis and TB were treated simultaneously. Same medicines were continued as long as there was improvement without any change in symptoms; when hepatitis improved, *Phos.* was given less frequently in higher potency and the frequency of *Sepia* was increased. Change in symptoms and signs (abdomen pain and fluid in the pouch of Douglas) led to a change in medicine (*Bry.* and *Thuj.*). Remarkable improvement in the patient's health led to an ahead of schedule endometrial biopsy which showed absence of previously present *Mycobacterium tuberculosis.* It could be deemed to be the effect of antibiotics taken for about eleven weeks. Two thoughts struck me: since the action of these drugs is on the removal of bacteria only, then why should they be used for a longer period of time, causing a perceptible deterioration in the health of the patient? Second, it is also possible that simultaneous use of multiple indicated homeopathy remedies used frequently, complemented each other and led to the enhancement of endogenous immunological processes, causing complete annihilation of bacteria and speedy restoration of health. The complaint for which she had come to the infertility clinic was cured with the much simpler and smaller procedure of Intra Uterine Insemination (IUI) than the proposed In Vitro Insemination (IVF).*

Abdominal TB with intestinal obstruction

In April 2013, a case of abdominal TB with drug intolerance was referred to me for alternate treatment. The patient was a sixty-one-year-old lady, accompanied by an entourage of six men and another lady. All had incredulous expressions on their face—homeopathy in TB!! Never heard of!!!. But since allopathy was not suiting her, there was no other option.

The lady had been admitted into the emergency ward two days earlier for colicky abdominal pain, distension, vomiting, loose stools and queasiness of three days' duration. On the basis of a CECT, a CT scan of the abdomen on 28 March 2013, a positive Quantiferon TB Gold test on 29 March 2013 and two previous such episodes, conventional ATT with *Akt4* was prescribed on 29 March 2013. Twelve days later, she complained of similar symptoms and the treatment was stopped. Colonoscopy (Figure 5A, see p. 4 of insert) revealed lesions similar to TB, though a biopsy and polymerase chain reaction (PCR) test for *Mycobacterium tuberculosis* were negative. Liver function tests were within normal limits. *Akt4* restarted, but the patient's condition worsened after one week, along with further loss of weight.

---

*Published: Chand, K.S., 'Homeopathy in the Treatment of Tuberculosis', *AJHN*, Summer, 2013, vol. 102, no. 2.

I saw her at this point when the efforts of taking specific TB treatment (so-called) had failed. Homeopathic treatment started according to regime. *Lyc.*, one dose once in the morning, selected as patient-specific medicine for poor appetite and little food causing abdominal distension which became better by passing flatus. *Carb-v.*, one dose twice a day before lunch and dinner, was for distension of the abdomen better by eructation, indigestion from simplest food and as a complementary medicine to *Lyc. Tub.* was disease-specific nosode, one dose once a week. After a month, the pain and distension of abdomen was less and appetite had improved, but she complained of itching in the eyes, treated with addition of a few doses of *Ars*. On her third visit, she complained of nausea, acidity, stiffness of the leg, though she was eating well and gaining in weight. The prescription was changed to match the symptoms. Fourth time, the complaint of acidity was clearly due to overeating and indulgence in fried food, treated with *Puls*. She was advised to observe restraint and repeat the colonoscopy test. After three weeks there were no complaints. Colonoscopy (Figure 5B, see p. 4 of insert) showed complete healing of ulcers with a contracted caecum. Treatment was continued for another month. The patient continued to be well and without any recurrence till her last visit in November 2016.

Observation: This elderly patient had been suffering from abdominal symptoms for a few months. She had been admitted into the emergency twice earlier, managed empirically and discharged. Third time ATT was given on the basis of clinical experience and investigations. Patient was unable to continue the treatment, maybe because of summation of disease symptoms and drug effects. Colon biopsy was negative for *Mycobacterium tuberculosis*, though the lesions were similar to TB. The response to only homeopathy was not only symptomatic, but also curative as in complete healing of ulcers. Management of all unrelated symptoms like itchy eyes and stiffness of legs was under one roof.

It is possible that it was a case of paucibacillary TB which responded well to only homeopathy.[*]

Integration of homeopathy with allopathy from the beginning shortens treatment time

Pulmonary TB

Prem Kumar, a twenty-four-year-old chauffeur of a doctor friend, was sent on 1 April 2020 for the treatment of cough with scanty expectoration, mild fever and loss of weight of one month's duration. He had a history of a disturbed family life. Radiograph of the chest showed prominent hilar shadows and right-sided bilateral fibrotic lesions (Figure 6, see p. 4 of insert), but the sputum smear was negative for *Mycobacterium tuberculosis,* also known as Acid Fast Bacillus (AFB). On the basis of prolonged fever, loss of weight and chest radiograph, clinical diagnosis of pulmonary TB was made and simultaneously, allopathic ATT was started. On first consultation for homeopathy, a dose of *Dros.* was given for the cough which caused a rise in the fever. This was addressed first with *Puls.* on the indication of an afternoon rise of temperature accompanied with sleepiness followed by chill at 4 pm. When it abated to mild fever, regimen

---

[*]Published by Chand, K.S., Kapoor, P. 'Case reports on integrated management of tubercular disease', *Homeopathy*, 2017, 106 (2), 214–22.

treatment began. *Phos.* was the patient-specific medicine on the basis of cough aggravated by lying on the left side and grief of a disturbed family life ruining health; it was complemented with *Sulph., Ars-i.* was given for mediastinal lymphadenopathy and cachexia, *Ip.* for nausea and a weekly dose of *Tub.* as disease-specific medicine. The patient improved progressively in all parameters with this combined plan of treatment. After two months, he complained of painful swelling of the knee and ankle joints and stiffness of legs. This was due to an increased level of uric acid. This was managed by withdrawing of *Pyrazinamide* (one of the drugs in *Akt4)* and change in homeopathic medicines from *Phos.* and *Ars.* to *Lyc.* and *Led. Tub.* continued as before.

Allopathic ATT was stopped after four and a half months, six weeks earlier than the prescribed time. Homeopathy continued for another month as a precaution. The recovery was smooth and permanent as the patient was closely followed for the next three years.

Observation: The experiment of combining two therapeutic systems was successful. It shortened the treatment period and reduced the intake of antibiotics.

Pleural effusion

A thirteen-year-old boy was referred on 16 January 2016 with the complaint of right-sided pleural effusion along with nausea, no appetite, epigastric pain, constipation and fever for one week. He had a history of upper respiratory tract allergy since he was ten years old. Conventional

---

*Published by Chand, K.S., Kapoor, P. 'Case reports on integrated management of tubercular disease', *Homeopathy*, 2017, 106 (2), 214–22.

ATT had been started a day earlier with advice to consult homeopathy for allergy and the psychiatry department for abdominal symptoms as the patient was a finicky eater and trembled from fear of being scolded. A homeopathic regime of medicine comprised of *Bry.* twice a day for fever, no appetite and white-coated tongue; *Kali-c.*, one dose twice a week on Tuesdays and Saturdays for abdominal complaints and pleural effusion; *Tub.*, one dose once a week on Sundays as disease-specific nosode. There was no fever after a week but other symptoms continued. He complained of vomiting after eating. The medicine was changed to *Calc-p.*, one dose once a week for easy vomiting, *Colch.* once a day for intense nausea from smell of food and pleural effusion; *Bry.* and *Tub.* continued as before. Two months later, the patient had no abdominal pain, was eating well and had gained weight; but complained of sneezing on swimming. He was given *Ars.* once in the morning and *Carb-v.* twice a day, *Tub.* continued as before. On 14 May 2016, the patient was asymptomatic, no pleural effusion, the slight blunting of the cost-phrenic angle was due to thickened pleura. All treatment was stopped.

Observation: Patient was on an integrated treatment from the beginning. He had many symptoms not directly related to the disease and strong respiratory allergy, but the recovery was steady and smooth. A comprehensive homeopathy regime cured allergy as well as psychiatric symptoms along with pleural effusion. The duration of conventional treatment was shortened by at least two months.

Addition of homeopathy potentiates the action of antibiotics

Pott's spine

After a clinical grand round meeting in the hospital in November 2014, a colleague asked me whether I had treated a case of TB spine, also known as Pott's spine. On affirming so, he shared with me the story of a young woman, suffering from this disease. She had been suffering from back ache for the last year and a half. The initial year had been spent in visiting various general practitioners (GPs), who had treated her with multiple pain-relieving drugs without any improvement. A simple radiograph of the spine had revealed nothing abnormal. Then she began to develop fever by the evening and a swelling appeared by the side of the upper part of the spine. A Magnetic Resonance Imaging (MRI) test revealed it to be a paravertebral abscess along with involvement of dorsal vertebrae (Figure 7, see p. 5 of insert). A clinical and radiological diagnosis of Pott's spine was made and ATT comprising five antibiotics with other adjuvant drugs started. 30 ml of pus was drained from the cold abscess and the patient discharged from the hospital with advice to use a Taylor's Brace for back support. Twelve days later, she was admitted again as a case of drug-induced gastritis with the inability to accept anything orally; liver enzymes were deranged, indicating hepatitis. She was put on intravenous fluids, drugs and 25 ml of pus drained again. She was discharged after two days with alternate anti-tubercular drugs. Patient was readmitted after a month with the same symptoms in increased intensity and loss of weight. Since there was no response to treatment and the patient was bedridden, two more opinions from specialists in two different hospitals were taken, who advised the same treatment. It was apparent that the disease had not responded to antibiotics, and the patient was advised to try homeopathy.

I saw her on 6 November 2014. She was looking toxic, running high fever, could hardly sit from pain and appeared to be in an advanced stage of disease. I was in a dilemma; homeopathy is considered to be a mild and gentle therapeutic system meant for treatment of symptoms and early-stage disease. After much thought, I made the full regime of homeopathy; but asked the father to give only one dose of one medicine in a day and continue with all the allopathic medicines. He was also told to report the outcome after five days. On the fifth day, he rang up to inform the downturn of fever and return of appetite. Pleasantly surprised, I told him to give the full homeopathy regime, along with allopathy. *Sulph. 30c* one dose in the morning on Tuesdays and Fridays, was selected as a patient-specific medicine for TB vertebrae, psoas abscess, inflammation of liver, nausea after eating, thirst for large quantities of water; *Symph. 30c* once in the morning on the other four days, as organ-specific medicine for caries of vertebra and psoas abscess; *Sil. 6c* twice a day as a general stimulant and for psoas abscess; *Ip. 6c* twice a day for constant nausea and hepatitis; *Tub. 200c* one dose once a week as disease-specific nosode.

On her second visit after three weeks, she had gained 2 kg in weight; the paravertebral swelling had markedly reduced in size and did not need draining. After seven weeks, on 27 December 2014, her general condition had improved to the extent that she was able to move around and manage herself, but complained of painful stiffness of back, more so in the lower part. X-ray of the dorsal spine showed no evidence of bony trauma or lesion and paravertebral shadows were normal (Figure 8, see p. 6 of insert). The treating orthopaedic surgeon and the gastroenterologist were amazed at the outcome and left the choice of continuing antibiotics with us. The X-ray and MRI of the spine were not comparable, but, since there was remarkable improvement in general health, and going by our previous experience, allopathy was stopped as it had been given for fourteen weeks. Homeopathy continued for further eleven months with changes according to symptoms and MRI reports.

Observation: Seven weeks of bacteria-specific antibiotics had had no effect on the disease. Addition of patient-specific homeopathy had a remarkable curing effect. I presumed the combination potentiated the anti-bacterial effect of antibiotics. Total duration of allopathy was only fourteen weeks, as against the minimum of nine to twelve months.

Multidrug-resistant pulmonary TB

This case was referred by a homeopath who had heard my talk on 'Integrated treatment in tubercular disease'. The patient was a young married lady who had been suffering for two years. The disease which began with a cough and rise of fever in the evenings was diagnosed on chest radiography as right-sided pleural effusion. After ten months of ATT treatment, the pleural effusion had improved, leaving behind a thick layer of liquid; though the fever and cough continued. The advice of surgical removal of the thick layer was ignored because of the forthcoming marriage of

---

*Published by Chand, K.S., Kapoor, P. 'Case reports on integrated management of tubercular disease', *Homeopathy*, 2017, 106 (2), 214–22.

the patient. Instead, she was treated by another specialist, whose non-ATT treatment led to increase in weight by 5 kg. The family relaxed as increase in weight is one of the important parameters of wellness in TB, and ignored the continued dry cough and mild fever. After marriage, the intensity of fever increased gradually and she had to be admitted in hospital. A computerized tomography (CT) scan of the chest showed pleural effusion and partial collapse of the lung, which were deemed to be the sequelae of the previous disease. Since the Widal test for typhoid was also positive, she was treated with suitable antibiotics for typhoid, but the fever continued with the same intensity. She was reinvestigated for TB. Reports of sputum culture and the Gene test were positive for AFB and DST confirmed MDR TB. ATT was started with one injectable and four oral antibiotics, along with adjuvant medicines. Six weeks of this treatment gave no symptomatic relief in fever, cough with profuse expectoration, nausea, vomiting and aversion to food.

Homeopathic help was sought at this point for symptomatic relief. It was added to allopathic treatment, with weekly doses of constitutional medicine *Phos.*, and its complementary *Sulph.*, disease-specific *Tub., Ferr-p.* for fever, *Sang.* for cough with expectoration. After a week, the vomiting had stopped and the fever showed a downward trend.

After one month, the continuous cough was absent during the day. The patient had a cough after eating/ taking medicine, purulent expectoration at 3 am during the night and a sensation of a lump in her throat. She complained of attacks of profuse sweating with weakness and dizziness and no appetite in the morning. *Kali-c.* was added once in the morning for four days of the week, and *China.+ Sang.* was given once in evening every day. The rest of the medicines continued as before. Except for a weekly dose of disease-specific *Tub.*, other medicines were reassessed on every monthly visit and changed according to prominent presenting symptoms. There was gradual improvement in symptoms. Fever was first to go after four months, then cough and expectoration, weakness, and menses appeared after eight months. The increase in weight was observed after a continuous fall for the first six months. There was improvement in the chest radiograph after two months and a remarkable improvement at seven months, which continued (Figure 9, see p. 6 of insert).

The injectable antibiotic was withdrawn after two months because of dizziness. Others were withdrawn after sixteen and a half months as against twenty-four months.

Observation: The first round of ATT for ten months did not cure the disease completely; the patient continued to have fever and cough. Maybe she had MDR TB since the beginning, which was later proved with Gene, culture and drug-sensitivity tests. Six weeks of second-generation ATT drugs given to MDR TB patients had no effect, actually her general condition had worsened. This led them to seek alternate treatment with homeopathy. The response to combined treatment with the same antibiotics was curative. The patient slowly and progressively improved, and amenorrhoea of eight months was also cured without addition of hormones.

Homeopathy in recurrent disease

On a cold January morning in 2018, a patient was announced in my hospital chamber. I raised my head and saw a familiar-looking elderly lady. Before I could place her, she heaved a sigh of relief and said, 'Thank God, you are there,' meaning 'you are alive'. By that time, I had placed her as case no. 15 in the tubercular project. I was seeing her after fifteen years. She had come with the complaint of recurrent cervical lymphadenopathy. The present episode had recurred for the fifth time and she was being treated with six second-generation anti-tubercular antibiotics for the past three weeks without much improvement. She was very anxious and despaired about recovery. She had made her family actively seek my whereabouts for homeopathic intervention. The history of illness was disturbing; the first episode of illness had occurred in the year 2004. It was diagnosed as tubercular cervical lymphadenopathy (case no. 15) in the article published in the journal *Homeopathy* and was treated with Cat III ATT (irregular course due to adverse drug reactions) which improved the symptoms of weight loss and fever initially, but the sensation of weakness and enlarged lymph nodes persisted. This was followed with homeopathy at our project on TB in NHMC, with about three months of treatment. Her weakness had greatly improved and the lymph nodes had become impalpable. Next year, the same lymph nodes had increased again. The FNAC report showed granulomatous lymphadenitis but there were no other symptoms. She did not visit us again and the records of treatment were vague. The patient claimed to have taken homeopathy, possibly self-treatment based on previous prescriptions. The third episode occurred in 2009, with the same cervical lymph nodes, enlarged with an abscess, and all the previous subjective symptoms. The active job of being a principal of a school with irregular and poor eating habits was deemed to be the cause of recurrence. This time, the abscess was drained and ATT (*Akt4*) was taken for one year as advised. The fourth recurrence was in December of 2012 in the same area of the cervical region. It was treated with ATT for nine months, but there was no change in the lesion. A senior chest specialist from Ganga Ram hospital was consulted. Pus smear and culture/sensitivity tests showed the presence of *Burkholderia cepacia,* but since rapid AFB culture and accuprobe-culture-identification ruled out the presence of AFB, this infection was treated with a combination of broad-spectrum antibiotics for ten days without effect. An ultrasound of the neck showed multiple lymph nodes of various sizes with evidence of calcification and liquefaction necrosis. On a diagnosis of MDR TB, a regime of six ATT drugs, including injections of *Streptomycin,* was prescribed for a further eighteen months, which was meticulously adhered to in spite of adverse drug reactions.

The present episode happened in August 2017, after retirement when the patient was leading a relaxed and regular life. This caused a lot of anxiety. The advice to start ATT was refused and she was extensively investigated for malignancy/lymphoma. Mammography and extensive biochemical tests were within normal limits. The FNAC on 29 August 2017 of the right cervical lymph node was consistent with chronic narcotizing suppurative granulomatous inflammation; Gene expert test showed a *Mycobacterium tuberculosis* complex detected with low resistance to *Rifampicin*; she was put on *Akt4* from 22 December 2017.

Homeopathy treatment started from 13 January 2018

with *Bar-c. Sil.* and *Tub*. This was based on the symptoms: feverish feeling in the mornings and evenings, stiffness in the cervical region, absent/unsatisfactory stool, desire for hot drinks, mutton and sweets and past history/family history (sister) of TB, palpable lymph node, 1.5 cm, in right supraclavicular region, immobile, adherent to overlying skin and tender. She was reviewed every two weeks. On her second visit, *Carb-a.* was added for indurated glands in an old woman with low vitality. Allopathic treatment with antibiotics continued and six weeks later, she complained of lack of appetite and a sinking sensation. *Sil.* was replaced with *Puls.* Her symptoms progressively improved and the lymph nodes became very small in size. Antibiotics were stopped after three and a half months but homeopathy continued. The patient was hypochondriacal about the presence of lymph nodes, however small, hence the prescription changed to *Calc-i., Tub.* and *Sil. 6c.* After three months, the patient was convinced of the absence of lymph nodes, but had a fear of an incurable disease, which was cured with daily doses of *Ars.* for a month.

Observation: Patient suffered from recurrent disease in spite of meticulous adherence to treatment which was directed to control/eradiate the bacteria. The antibiotics led to a paucibacillary state, but could not control immune-pathology. Also a prolonged intake of antibiotics had lowered her vitality. Homeopathy improved immunity and controlled mental anxiety. There has been no recurrence till date.

PART SIX

The Way Forward

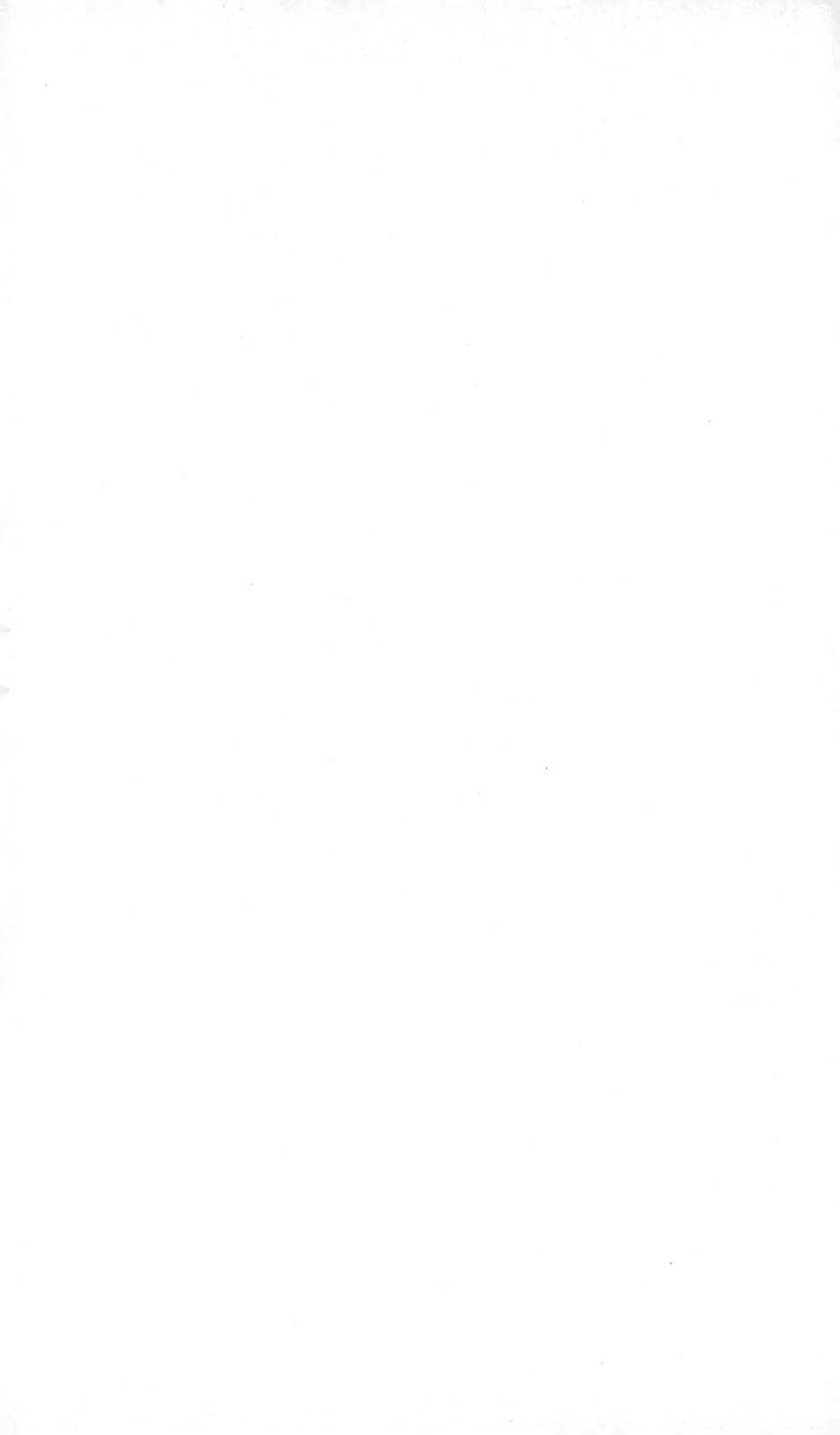

Twenty-one

Immunity, Disease and Medicine

In the flu epidemic of 1968, my seventy-year-old grandmother fell sick with cold, cough and mild fever; we were worried and anxious because of her age, but fortunately she recovered soon. Next to follow was her husband, who took longer to recover, though the disease was not severe; in my mind, I dismissed it as a desire to be pampered. Thereafter, one of my cousins, a young healthy girl in her early twenties of anxious temperament and poor eating habits, had a severe episode with high-grade fever and pneumonia. Her brother also had pneumonia, but recovered faster. The mother and another brother were not affected. I, as a young doctor focused only on the virus, was perplexed; six people living in the same environment get infected with the same virus at the same time, but respond so differently. There was something more than the virus to cause this response. The same response was observed during the current Covid-19 pandemic. By now I have greater knowledge of immunity and the homeopathic concept of disease, which I would like to share with my readers.

All living beings differ from the non-living by possessing a powerful self-defence mechanism. This is something by which any living cell, tissue or body responds to all external stimuli, beneficial or malefic. It can be defined as a complex biological system endowed with the capacity to recognize and tolerate whatever belongs to the self and reject what is foreign (non-self). In a human being, it comprises the immune system, the sympathetic and parasympathetic system, the hormonal system and much more.

It acts all the time and keeps the functions of the living being within the normal level of homeostasis. When it is healthy and intact, no change in health is evident. A robust immune system can overcome any virus/bacteria, while a weak immune system gets easily overwhelmed, leading to recurrent/continuous suffering. It also does not remain constant throughout life; it waxes and wanes with various physical or emotional stresses.

Malefic external agents are many; can be a microbe: virus, bacteria, fungus; environmental: change in weather or temperature; pollen; emotions; stress: mental/physical. When the malefic force is more powerful than the defence mechanisms, there is a change in health. More often, it is a combination of forces, where the microbe is the important immediate cause, though not the only cause.

There is a time lag between the attack by malefic forces and the appearance of the symptoms of the disease. This is called the latent period, during which defence mechanisms are reacting with the malefic forces, to arrive at a new level of homeostasis. This change in health is called disease: ill-at-ease. This may be expressed by symptoms at physical, emotional or mental level/levels. The totality of symptoms is the expression of the sick person with the disease and not the symptoms of a disease caused by a particular microbe.

Such a sick person may need help of an expert

(physician) to overcome the suffering caused by a new level of homeostasis. He/she does it with the help of medicine, which is the science and art dealing with the maintenance of health and the prevention, alleviation, or cure of disease. There are many modes of therapy which can alleviate human suffering. Each therapy has been dominant at some point in time in the history of mankind. Each one has its sphere of maximum action. To label one as the panacea of all diseases is a narrow-minded approach.

Homeopathy is focused on the teleonomy of the patient's reaction; it boosts the immunity; it would be more suitable in the early functional stage of a disease, when symptoms are many and structural changes are few/none. Hence it is suitable for general/family practice, where one tends to see patients in an early stage. It may particularly be suitable for children for its gentle, quick action and easy compliance. As immediate cause is taken lightly, in serious infections, total reliance on only homeopathy could worsen the condition of the patient and prolong the suffering.

Allopathy is focused on an immediate external cause, which is a microbe, thus immunity is taken for granted. In serious infections, when the causative microbe and the anti-microbial agent are known, allopathy will get prompt results. But empirical and prolonged use of antibiotics/antiviral drugs could be harmful, as the low immunity of the patient is further compromised with side-effects of the drugs leading to more serious chronic diseases.

A pre-designed basic homeopathic protocol helped me serve my society to the best of my capabilities even during the pandemic. This homeopathic regime worked broadly as a preventive and another one was designed for treatment during mild and moderate Covid-19 infections. In post-

Covid-19 syndromes, both mental and physical health were also addressed with homeopathic regimes. When there was scarcity of medicine, when hospital infrastructures had collapsed and there was shortage of all other drugs, many resorted to homeopathy for antiviral immune modulation. Studies done by the Central Council for Research in Homoeopathy (CCRH) have proved that the complementary use of these remedies contributed to reduce the duration of illness. I personally experienced this in my patients.

My experiments and experiences have shown that homeopathy and allopathy are complementary. Complementary use of homeopathy with allopathic antibiotics reduces recovery time, morbidity and increases drug compliance. It can be helpful in MDR TB and drug-intolerant cases. Experiments show that homeopathic medicines, when given in a regime form give reproducible results. The regime is patient-specific, targeting all the sufferings at the same time and is guided by the symptoms of the patient. The regime consists of a symptom-specific medicine targeting location of disease and presenting symptoms; a constitutional medicine based on physical and mental generals of the patient and a disease-specific nosode.

In the cure of chronic disease, different therapies are needed at different stages of the disease. None can be fully effective in relieving all aspects and stages of the disease. Often there is no molecular or genetic explanation justifying an increase of susceptibility to infection. The immediate cause could be microbial, but it is also true that the whole 'terrain' plays an important role in the expression of a disease. Both systems can be effectively used simultaneously for the benefit of the patient. The combined effect reduces morbidity and expedites recovery, more so in the management of chronic disease and recurrent infections. Of course, this requires a thorough knowledge of the pathology behind the disease and action of each medicine. When the microbial load is high, antibiotics are required. In recurrent infections, where the patient's immunity (reactive modalities) is low, homeopathy is more helpful. This is seen in chronic infections; if a patient is not responding to antibiotics, addition of suitable homeopathy leads to improvement with the same antibiotics.

Twenty-two

My Dream

WHO report on World TB Day, 2021

Each year, we commemorate World Tuberculosis (TB) Day on 24 March to raise public awareness about the devastating health, social and economic consequences of TB, and to step up efforts to end the global TB epidemic. The date marks the day in 1882 when Dr Robert Koch announced that he had discovered the bacterium that causes TB, which opened the way towards diagnosing and curing this disease.

TB remains one of the world's deadliest infectious killers. Each day, nearly 4000 lose their lives to TB and close to 28,000 people fall ill with this preventable and curable disease. Global efforts to combat TB have saved an estimated 63 million lives since the year 2000.

*The theme of World TB Day 2021—'**The Clock Is Ticking**'—conveys the sense that the world is running out of time to act on the commitments made by global leaders to end TB. This is especially critical in the context of the Covid-19 pandemic that has put End TB progress at risk, and to ensure equitable access to* *prevention and care in line with WHO's drive towards achieving Universal Health Coverage. The major limitations of allopathic TB treatment are increasing incidences of multidrug-resistant strains due to non-adherence to treatment leading to suboptimal response (failure and relapse); continuous spread of the disease, adverse drug events, co-infection of TB and HIV. The treatment of MDR TB with second-line drugs is very expensive, less potent, highly toxic, and of long duration (24–27 months); adherence to a regime is a major challenge. The optimal drug regimens are poorly characterized, and no fixed-dose combination tablets are in existence.*

There is no gold standard diagnostic test and treatment strategy for Latent TB Infection (LTBI) cases and it is expected that enormous numbers of new cases will arise, which will complicate the TB disease control programme. The Bacillus Calmette–Guérin (BCG) vaccine achieves early containment of *Myobacterium tuberculosis* in lesions and prevents severe disease in children, but is ineffective in long-term control, as it fails to eradicate the pathogen. Hence, it is questionable whether a vaccine that fails to achieve sterile eradication is sufficient.

So what needs to be done? The answer is not blowing in the wind, but in the hands of governments across the globe, as well as corporates and individuals invested in bringing the world closer to eradicating this disease.

While high-level pledges and sufficient funds are critical for an accelerated response to TB, two key multicomponent actions need to happen on the ground. There is a possibility to contribute to public health with a clear and focused strategy. Networks and collaborations must be developed. We should concentrate on well-established treatment strategies and explore the potential of constitutional treatment in multimorbid patients, treating people as individuals with complex health problems, not as multiple diseases each to be treated with different, and often multiple, drugs.

My experiences and experiments of over two decades, have convinced me of the usefulness of homeopathy in the management of TB. Medical pluralism is a unique feature of the Indian healthcare system and homeopathy is the second-most popular system in India. Its infrastructure includes 234 hospitals, 5910 dispensaries, 217,860 registered practitioners and 182 colleges. With such an infrastructure already in place, the two therapeutic systems can be easily implemented. This will lead to shorter duration of antibiotics, less adverse effects and more compliance.

Twenty-three

In Conclusion

Medicine has been practised since prehistoric times, during most of which it was an art (an area of skill and knowledge) frequently having connections to the religious and philosophical beliefs of a local culture. For example, a medicine man would apply herbs and say healing prayers, or an ancient philosopher and physician would apply bloodletting according to the theories of humourism. In recent centuries, since the advent of modern science, most medicine has become a combination of art and science (both basic and applied, under the umbrella of medical science). Pre-scientific forms of medicine are now known as traditional medicine or 'folk medicine', which remains commonly used in the absence of scientific medicine and are thus called alternative medicine.

My understanding of medicine has been evolving every day since I started my practice of medicine. Strict clinical diagnosis and specific allopathic medication was the mainstay of my prescription in the early years of practice. The constant need to search for disease reversal or functional medicine made me drift towards the homeopathic system of treatment. Managing multimorbid and complex cases led me to look for a middle way and the gap was bridged when I started getting long-term results from the integrated management of chronic patients. Every decade of clinical practice has made me believe that what is food for one could be medicine for someone else. What is prayer for one, could be medicine for someone else. What is fasting for one, could be detoxification for others. Laughter, sleep, friends, positivity, fearlessness, unconditional love, sharing, human touch and acceptance were raised to the pedestal of medicine worldwide during the Covid pandemic. We became aware of how vulnerable the human species is and how our immune system is choosing to fight strongly if it is stimulated in the right direction. To me homeopathy does this best and can be tailor-made to suit individual needs. Anti-microbial resistance is the next global pandemic. Are we ready to face it? Will there be any drug sensitivity for common microbes in the coming decades? How many and how effective new drugs can we develop to combat the menace of drug resistance? Can we look towards alternative therapies for the answer?

My main aim in writing this book is to create public and medical interest in seeking support from a qualified homeopath for recurrent infections and undiagnosed cases where symptoms are many but reports are normal. Let us use homeopathy as preventive medicine, for this is where homeopathy works best, a point where lifestyle measures have failed and the system is dodging towards instability or disease. Once a disease is established deeper and drug effects have caused complex disease patterns, let's think of integrating this nano-medicine to promote disease reversal if possible. The journey has just begun. The road less taken is where I walked for years, lonely at times but never disheartened. The constant experimentation with my homeopathic remedies in a variety of disease conditions always gave me a sound night's sleep and enough motivation to explore the scope of homeopathy in the next difficult case. My work is an offering to any doctor seeking similar satisfaction and to any patient wanting to turn to these pills for support. To me medicine is hope that we must give to each patient we encounter.

Experiments with drugs diluted to an unbelievable extent have been effective in relieving the suffering of the patient, without adding the burden of adverse drug reactions. The improvement has been subjective and objective, quick and gentle. Sometimes, when we can't explain a phenomenon or an observation, we either tend to ignore it, or call it a stray incident or magic. As science provides a solution and a rationale for everything, the scientific-minded person calls it unscientific. If there is anything that appears like a miracle, the only explanation is that a scientific reason for it has not been discovered as yet. From the intellectualist and functionalist perspectives, magic is often considered most analogous to science and technology.

Anything that helps the patient in recovering from disease is medicine. It should not be judged by its size, but by its effect. If a benevolent smile or compassionate words to a lonely person or homeopathy pills can help the patient, then why use the drugs which are potentially harmful.

This work is no claim to the scientific validity of homeopathy. At the same time, the clinical outcomes are irrefutable. The theory of the placebo effect, doctor's demeanour and the time spent on history is effectively countered.

The final validation from quantum physics is awaited. It will come. After all it took 400 years for Pythagoras to prove that the earth is round rather than flat.

Acknowledgements

My deep gratitude goes to Satish for a meaningful togetherness of twenty-six years. As a husband, he steered me into what I am today. His idea of marriage meant 'being together', making me resign from a lucrative job in anatomy that resulted in my becoming the physician that I am today.

As a doctor, I kept my passion for medicine alive within the framework of a joint family. 'Family first' has been my guiding star. Since I was not looking for any monetary or positional gains from medicine, it helped me see the shortcomings of allopathy. So, thank you to the Indian joint family system; and my parents' progressive attitude in educating a girl child within it.

I am thankful to Suresh for introducing me to his elite group of allopath friends and to the entire group for graciously embracing me as part of the group.

My gratitude goes to Dr Raj K. Manchanda for inducting me into the government's project on tuberculosis and giving me a free hand to experiment. Thanks also to the team of five senior research officers: Dr Anjali Miglani for her sincere work; Dr Sudhir Batra for his meticulous initial analysis of the huge data and Dr Renu Mittal for her final analysis, which were invaluable. Thank you, Dr Priya Kapoor, for your persuasive prodding to write this book, and Ruby Bansal for referring HIV cases for integrated treatment.

This work could not have taken the form of a book without Lakshmi. I have no words to thank her, but can only be a proud mother. Thank you, Divya for being my first sounding board, and Anju for patiently assisting me in writing the non-medical part of the book and sequencing the medical case-histories. Ever-ready Anu has been prompt in extending help whenever needed, which was often. Thanks to Ram, Rahoul, Anoushka and Ojaswita for their useful suggestions.

Thanks to my editor, Aruna Ghosh. You have done a great job of keeping my voice intact while making a medical chronicle enjoyable for the lay reader. Thank you, Renuka and Speaking Tiger for publishing the book. I appreciate your team for their compassionate handling of all my quirky requests.

Last but not the least: A big thank you to family, friends and to ALL those, who 'dared' to be treated by me, for nearly five decades. Each one has added to my learning and to the book.

APPENDIX

Case Histories of Tuberculosis

Retrospective study of fifty cases of TBLN revealed that in twenty-five cases, the records were complete according to protocol: all the investigations, particularly the FNAC, were done either before or within fifteen days of starting the treatment. Follow-up of all cases till the end stage was available, in a few longer follow-up was also present.

The summary of these cases of TBLN giving details of onset and duration of disease, investigations, selection of remedies from the individualized repertory graph (RG), duration and outcome of treatment is given below.

The cases have been placed in chronological order to highlight the evolution of the treatment regimen.

1. 08/21/2000 to 04/16/01

RM, 15 yrs, Hindu working as a helper at a restaurant.

He complained of gradually increasing swellings in the right groin for 12 months and frequent attacks of cold and cough since childhood. No history of taking conventional ATT.

O/E Small-built with pale waxy face, dull, indifferent to disease, easily tired, profuse perspiration at night and on least exertion and desire for eggs; 3 enlarged inguinal lymph nodes on right side, 1–2

Appendix: Case Histories of Tuberculosis

x 3 cm, painless, matted, not adherent to overlying skin. FNAC (08/21/2000) showed 'Tuberculous lymphadenitis in a reactive background'. Chest X-ray (No. 1516) (07/31/2000) 'Left hilum nodular, Lungs clear.' Hb.-9.2 gm%, TLC-6500, P60, L35, E04, M01, ESR-50 mm.

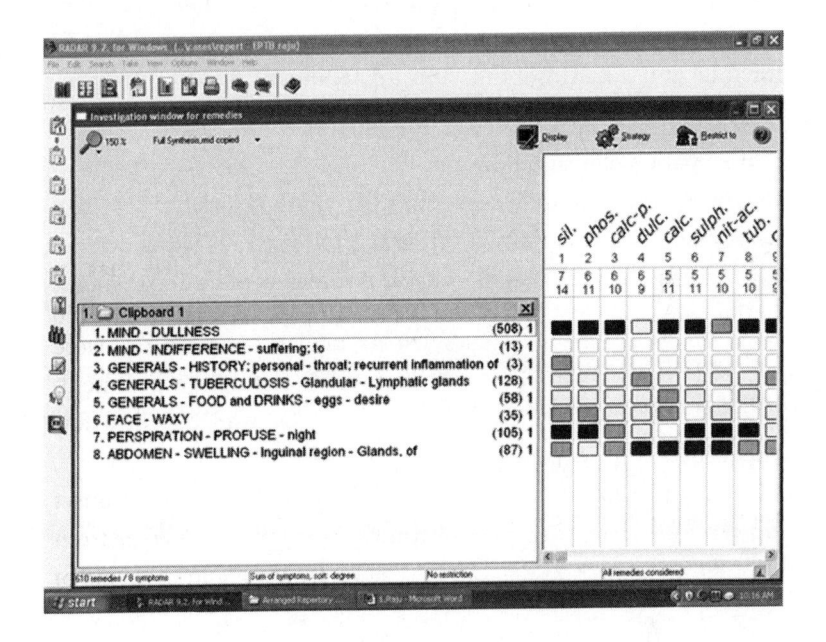

R was prescribed *Sil. 200c* tds once every 15 days and *Sil. 6D* tds for 14 days on 08/21/2000. *Tub. 200c*, one dose was added twice in 6 months, when the progress became static.

The lymph nodes progressively decreased in size to less than 1 x 1 cm in 8 months time. Hb 13.5 gm/dl, TLC 5,400, P65, L32, E02, M01, ESR 15 mm, chest X-ray (560) was normal on 04/16/01, weight gain of 4 kg.

Observations: Sil. 200c was the constitutional, globally indicated remedy selected on repertorization of all the presenting symptoms. *Sil. 6D* was used as a stimulant to leucocytes for phagocytic and fibroblastic activity; *Tub. 200c* as an intercurrent nosode.

2. 08/16/2001 to 07/22/02

S, 24 yrs, F, Hindu, housewife

S had gradually increasing swellings, pain and stiffness in the neck for the last three years. FNAC of the right cervical lymph node (03/19/2001): 'areas of necrosis in which numerous AFB are identified, compatible with Tuberculosis'; treated with ATT for four and a half months, stopped treatment due to intolerable gastrointestinal symptoms.

Homeopathic consultation on 08/16/01 for the complaints of weight loss of 4 kg in last five months, marked lassitude, vertigo, backache; pain in abdomen on eating followed by flatulence and sour eructations; cold hands and feet worse in winters and swellings in the neck

O/E group of 3–4 enlarged lymph nodes in the right anterior cervical region; matted together, 1 x 3 cm, not adherent to the overlying skin.

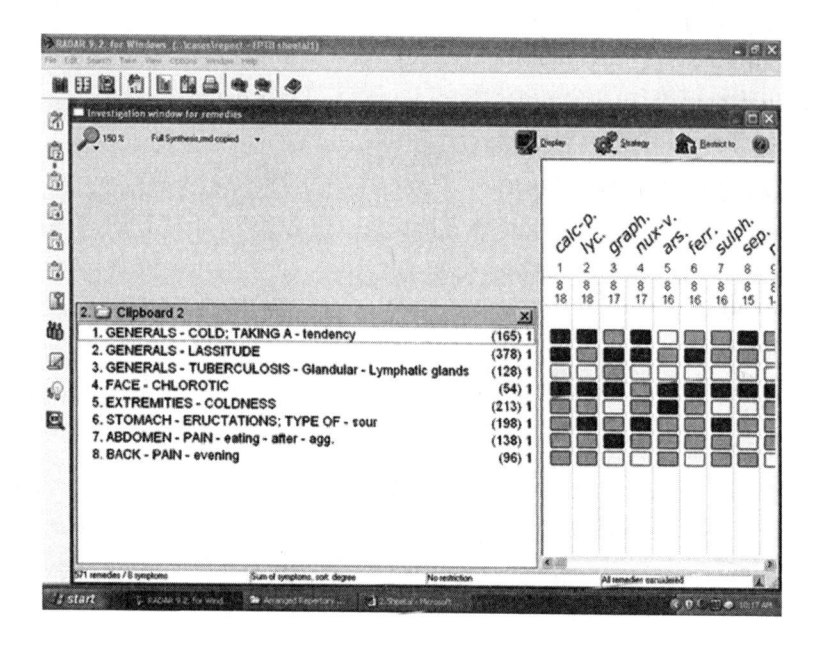

Investigations: On 08/16/2001; Hb.-9.2gm/dl,TLC-6800, P62, L36, E01, M01, ESR 38 mm, chest X-ray (No. 1456): 'Right paratracheal lymphadenopathy. Tubercular lesions seen in Left Upper Zone and mid zone.' Sputum smear and culture for AFB negative.

S's prominent presenting symptoms besides lymphadenopathy were stiffness of the neck, backache and cold extremities, hence treatment was started with *Calc-p*. *D6*, four times a day and *Tub*. *200c*, one dose once a month for initial two months. The initial response was slow improvement in general condition, backache, dyspeptic symptoms and in the size of lymph nodes but there was no change in cough, chest pain; she also had persistent thirst for very cold water, dry parched lips and stitching pain in chest. She even developed one new lymph node.

S was prescribed *Phos*. *30c* and *Tub*. *200c*, one dose every 15th day (alternately) and *Calc-p*. *D6* tds on 12/27/01.

The symptoms and the size of the lymph nodes progressively reduced in next three months and became less than 1 x 1 cm. The subsequent chest X-ray done on 07/22/02 (No. 1913) was normal, but for opacity in the mid zone indicative of old healed lesion. Hb increased to 12 gm/dl and ESR reduced to 20 mm, weight gain of 5 kg. Total duration of treatment was 11 months.

Observation: AFB positive lymphadenitis did not respond to four and a half months of ATT, patient had to stop treatment due to intolerable adverse drug effects and worsening of general condition. With homeopathy she completed the treatment without any adverse drug effects; was asymptomatic with marked reduction in the size of lymph nodes.

176 Appendix: Case Histories of Tuberculosis

3. 10/31/01 to 03/07/02

A, 8 yrs, M, Hindu.

A complained of gradually increasing swellings on both sides of the neck, breathlessness on exertion and dry cough for 4 months, frequent attacks of cold and cough and loose motions since childhood. History of PTB in grandfather.

O/E fair, fat and sweaty child with pale face, enlarged bilateral lymph nodes like knotted cords, painless, firm, 0.5–2.0 cm, not adherent to the overlying skin.

Investigations: On 10/31/01: FNAC 'Granulomatous lesion with caseating necrosis, no AFB seen', Hb.-10.6 gm/dl, TLC-7500, DLC -P46, L50, E04, ESR 38 mm, chest X-ray showed 'hilar lympadenopathy'.

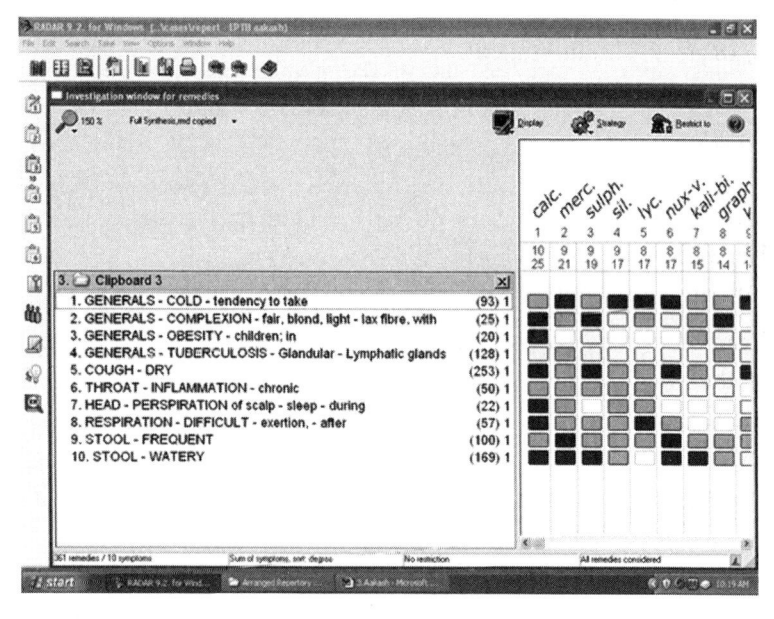

A was prescribed *Calc. 30c* tds x 1 day a wk on 10/31/01.

Symptoms improved in 2 months by 12/28/01, but the lymph nodes stopped reducing in size, then *Tub. 200c* x 1 dose a wk and

Sil. 6D tds for 5 days a wk was added. The size of the lymph nodes progressively reduced over a period of 3 months. Investigations on 03/07/02: Hb 12.1gm/dl, TLC 6,400, P63 L30 E04 M03; ESR 21 mm; chest X-ray showed hilar lymphadenopathy which was less as compared to previous X-ray.

Follow-up: 15 months, when he was treated with homeopathy for various ailments like pyoderma, cold and cough, chest pain and headache.

Observations: Patient was fully treated with only homeopathy during and after the disease. With *Calcarea carbonica* there was complete amelioration of symptoms, but the lymph nodes regressed only partially; addition of *Sil.* and *Tub.* completed the cure.

4. 05/27/02 to 10/13/03

L, 18 yrs, F, Hindu, student.

L suffered from abdomen TB one year ago, treated with Cat I ATT for 6 months (complete course) and was cured of the abdominal complaints. Soon after, she noticed the development of gradually increasing hard swellings in the right axillary and cervical region. Her father had died of PTB the previous year and brother was suffering from depression.

L came for homeopathic consultation on 04/30/02 for the treatment of the swellings and symptoms like breathlessness and pain in chest, worse on lying down; headache, more on right temporal region, better by pressure and by closing the eyes; had the fear that something bad will happen; desired and felt better in company, felt anxious about her family; had aversion for milk and fat, preferred salty food.

O/E enlarged lymph nodes on the right side, 2 in the axillary and 1 in the anterior cervical region, each about 2 x 2 cm, painless, hard and mobile.

Appendix: Case Histories of Tuberculosis

Investigations: On 04/30/02: FNAC 'Tuberculous lymphadenitis, no AFB seen,' Hb.-10 gm/dl, TLC-8,000, P62, L34, E02, M02, ESR-55 mm, chest X-ray (1515) normal.

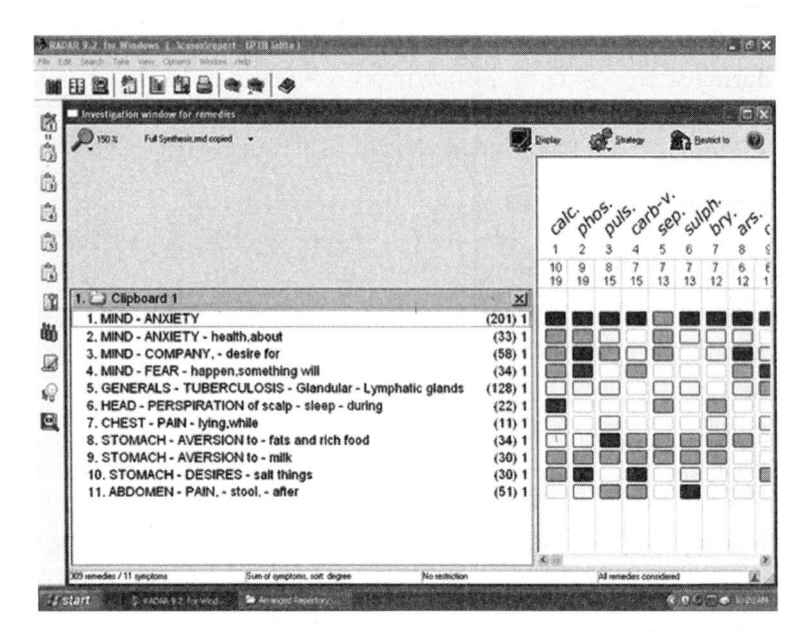

L was given *Phos. 30c* x 1 dose on 04/30/02. After initial improvement, she complained of feverish feeling and weakness, with no change in previous symptoms on 06/03/02. It was found that she had profuse sweat on head while sleeping. *Calc. 30c* x 1 dose every 15 days was prescribed.

The patient steadily and slowly improved in all the symptoms. One dose of *Tub. 200c* was added twice as an intercurrent medicine whenever the improvement stopped. The lymph nodes markedly reduced in size and consistency along with amelioration of all the associated symptoms in 17 months' time. Hb 12gm/dl, TLC 7600, P67 L30 E01 M02 ESR 20 mm on 10/13/03.

Observations: Patient developed tubercular lymphadenopathy, cough with anorexia and weight loss six months after a complete course of conventional ATT for PTB. There was complete amelioration in symptoms (subjective improvement) and marked reduction in the size of lymph nodes (objective improvement) with homeopathy. *Phos.* and *Calc.* had equal points on repertorization, but *Phosphorus* did not cover two symptoms, perspiration of scalp during sleep and chest pain on lying down, hence it wasn't the correct similimum.

5. 04/30/02 to 02/24/03

G, 28 yrs, M, Hindu, rickshaw driver from very poor strata.

G was diagnosed as a case of PTB one year ago, treated with Cat I ATT for 6 months, completed the treatment on 10/15/01. During next 6 months he developed swellings in the neck, cough with greyish sputum, more in the morning; breathlessness during cough; vertigo on standing; body aches; cramps during sleep; anorexia and loss of weight. He was referred to the chest clinic and came for homeopathic consultation on 04/30/02.

O/E 2 enlarged lymph nodes, one on each side in the anterior cervical area, 2 x 2.5 cm, painless, firm and mobile.

Investigations: (04/30/02) chest X-ray (1932) 'healed lesion in the left upper lobe with increased lung markings', sputum smear and culture negative, FNAC 'granulomatous lesion compatible with TB, no AFB seen.' Hb 9.0m/dl, TLC 12000, P58, L38, E4, MO, ESR 34 mm.

G was prescribed *Calc. 30c*, 1 dose once in 15 days.

There was gradual improvement in the symptoms, first in cough and expectoration then in appetite, the lymph nodes started decreasing after 3 months. Duration of treatment was 10 months with marked amelioration of symptoms, decrease in size of lymph nodes to less than 1 cm, Hb 11.5gm/dl, TLC 7,800, P62, L30, E 04, MO4, ESR 20 mm, increase in weight by 2 kg.

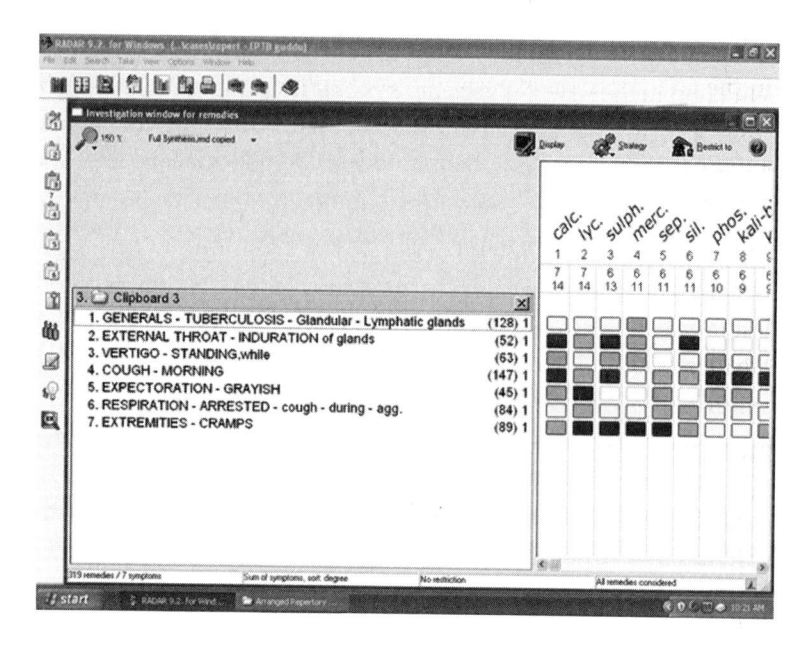

Observations: Patient developed tubercular lymphadenopathy, cough with anorexia and weight loss six months after a complete course of conventional ATT for PTB. There was first amelioration in symptoms (subjective improvement); reduction in the size of lymph nodes (objective improvement) began after three months of regular repetition of same medicine. The duration of treatment was long as classical method of one remedy at infrequent intervals was used.

6. 09/23/02 to 12/30/02

M, 7 yrs, M, Hindu.

M had prolonged fever with cough and expectoration at the age of 3 years. Since then, he has had frequent attacks of evening rise of temperature and cough with expectoration.

Homeopathic consultation on 09/23/02 for complaints of swellings in the neck for 4 years and dry hacking cough for 6 weeks, frequent hiccups, vomiting and loss of weight.

Appendix: Case Histories of Tuberculosis 181

O/E rough hands with cracked skin of the palms; cough aggravated in the afternoon, on exposure to cold and after eating; 1 enlarged right post auricular lymph node along with chain of bilateral anterior cervical group of lymph nodes, 0.5 to 2 cm, hard, discrete and mobile.

Investigations: (07/27/2002) chest X-ray (No. 2109) 'Left hilar lymph nodes ++. Lung parenchyma is clear.' FNAC 'granulomatous lesion with caseation necrosis consistent with TB, no AFB seen,' Hb10gm/dl, TLC 5900, P39, L46, E12, M3; ESR 65 mm, sputum smear negative for AFB.

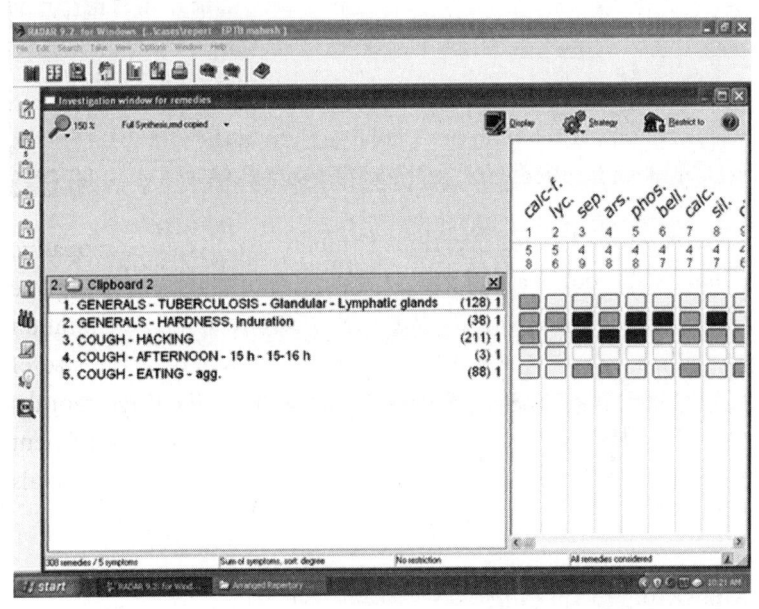

[Screenshot of RADAR 9.2 for Windows repertorization software showing:
2. Clipboard 2
1. GENERALS - TUBERCULOSIS - Glandular - Lymphatic glands (128) 1
2. GENERALS - HARDNESS, Induration (38) 1
3. COUGH - HACKING (211) 1
4. COUGH - AFTERNOON - 15 h - 15-16 h (3) 1
5. COUGH - EATING - agg. (88) 1

Remedies: calc-f., lyc., sep., ars., phos., bell., calc., sil.]

M was given *Tub. 200c,* 1 dose once a fortnight and *Calc-f. 6D* tds. Two bouts of fever were treated with *Puls. 30c* qid (fever at 2 pm, followed by chill at 4 pm and sweating at night, no thirst with dry lips).

The total duration of treatment was three months with lymph nodes less than 1 cm in size and no symptoms. Hb 12.5gm/dl, TLC 5400, P64, L28, E6, M2, ESR 22 mm.

Observation: This was the first patient treated with *Tub.* from the beginning, the indicated constitutional remedy was used in low decimal potency as recommended in Boericke's *Materia Medica*. The result was satisfactory without any aggravation.

7. 08/06/02 to 06/12/03

S, 5½ yrs, M, Hindu.

S was brought by his father on 08/06/02 for the complaints of swellings in the neck and dry cough of 3 months duration. History of frequent attacks of cold and cough particularly at the change of season and diarrhoea, father had PTB 10 yrs ago.

O/E small-built, pale child, easily tired on exertion with profuse sweating, bilateral lymph node enlargement in the anterior cervical region like a knotted cord, painless, 0.5 to 2.0 cm and mobile.

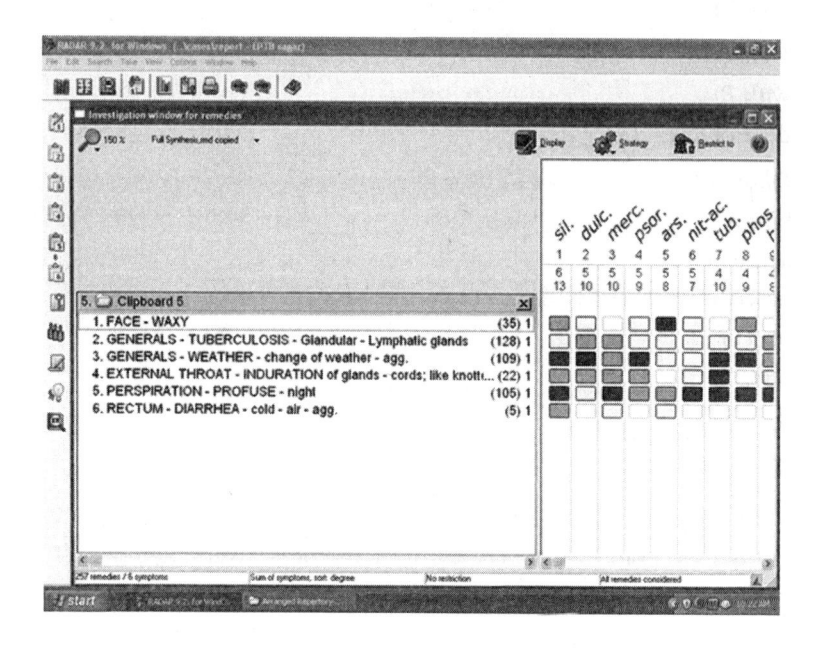

Investigations: (08/02/02) chest X-ray (310) 'nodular lung lesion seen in right upper lobe with prominent hilar shadow.'; FNAC 'granulomatous lymphadenitis, no AFB seen', Hb10.5gm/dl, TLC 6000, P28, L68, E4, MO, ESR 46 mm.

S was prescribed *Tub. 200c*, 1 dose once in 15 days, followed by *Sil. 6D* tds. *Sil. 200c*, 1 dose was given in the second week as a constitutional remedy. He developed an acute attack of cold in the winter with acrid nasal discharge, sneezing and feverishness, treated with *All-c. 30c* tds for 7 days, patient had developed moderate fever on 4th day; nasal discharge and sneezing became better but fever persisted on 8th day which was treated with *Ars. 30c* tds for 7 days. Then on a hot summer day, after playing outside in the park, he had a bath with cold water and suffered from an acute attack of nausea, vomiting and diarrhoea, effectively treated with *Ant-c. 30c* tds for 3 days.

S showed immediate improvement in cough and general condition, the lymph nodes started reducing after 4 months. Total duration of treatment was 10 months; after that only 3 lymph nodes remained of the size of less than 1 cm, Hb 12.5 gm/dl, TLC 7600, P36, L55, E04, M05, ESR 15 mm, weight gain by 1 kg.

Follow-up: Of 15 months. One episode of abdomen pain was treated with *Bry. 30c*, another of acute coryza with *Ars. 30c* followed by one dose of *Tub. 200c*.

Observation: Patient's treatment began with *Tub.* and *Sil.* based on family history of TB in father and patient's general condition. The acute episodes were treated with homeopathic-indicated medicine based on presenting symptoms. In the follow-up, giving a dose of *Tub.* after an episode of acute illness helped in recovery and reduced recurrence.

Patient was fully treated with only homeopathy including the acute episodes of coryza with fever and acute gastroenteritis.

8. 12/26/02 to 11/06/03

B, 5 yrs, M, Hindu.

The child was brought by the mother on 12/26/02 with the complaints of swellings in the neck noticed for 6 months which increased in last 2 months, accompanied by dry cough with scanty expectoration in the morning, aggravated on lying down, listless and feverish in the afternoon; no appetite and loss of weight. History of recurrent boils, PTB in grandmother.

O/E small-built, shy, weepy and clinging to the mother. Multiple enlarged lymph nodes on both sides of the neck like a knotted cord, 0.5 to 2.5 cm, matted, tender and firm, no fluctuation and mild fever.

Investigations: (12/26/02) chest X-ray (2450) 'right hilar lymph nodes enlarged, lung parenchyma normal.' FNAC 'granulomatous lesion consistent with tuberculosis, no AFB seen.' Hb.12 gm/dl, TLC 7500, P62, L33, E3, M2, ESR 62 mm.

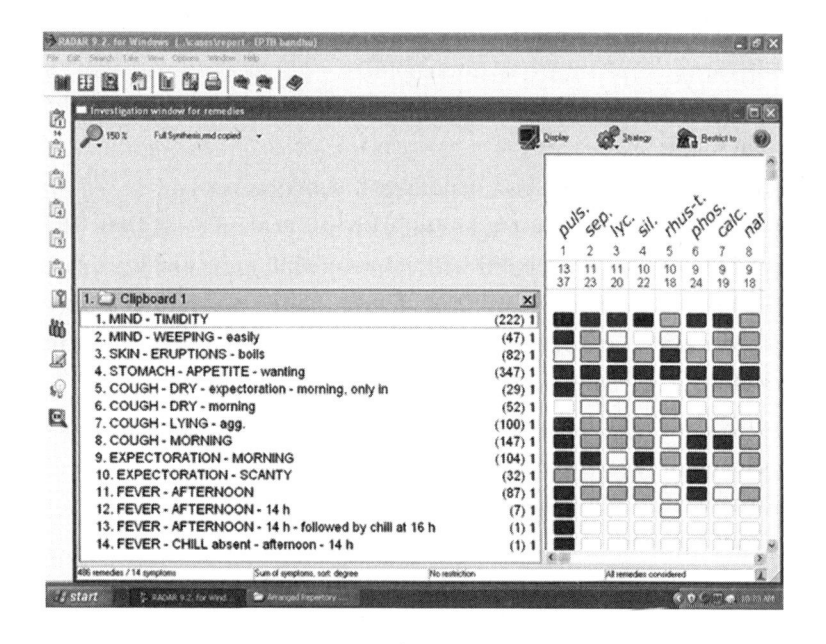

B was prescribed *Puls. 30c* tds x 2 wk on 12/26/02 for fever; no fever after 2 weeks, then treated with *Tub. 200c* x 1 dose once a fortnight and *Sil. 6D* tds. He had pyoderma on 07/24/03, which responded to the addition of weekly dose of *Staphyloc. 200c* for 3 weeks.

The response was good with amelioration of all the symptoms and most of the lymph nodes were impalpable, except one which regressed to less than 1 cm, soft in consistency. Duration of treatment was 11 months. Chest X-ray (3617) on 11/06/03 was better in comparison to previous report. Hb 13gm/dl, TLC 7000, P65, L25, E09, M01, ESR 32 mm.

Observation: This patient's treatment began by managing the fever with indicated homeopathic medicine before prescribing for enlarged lymph nodes. Treatment of pyoderma with indicated medicine resulted in smooth recovery.

9. 01/30/03 to 10/16/03

B, 17 yrs, M, Muslim, residing in a crowded area of the city.

B came to the general homeopathic outpatient department on 01/16/03 for the treatment of painful swelling in the neck, pain in chest and breathlessness of 6 weeks duration; had acute bronchitis 14 weeks ago, treated by allopathic physician, no ATT was given. The profuse expectoration had reduced but he developed breathlessness and pain in chest on coughing and exertion, chest X-ray (2860) 'there is a linear opacity along Right Lateral Chest Wall suggestive of pleural thickening.' He was referred to the chest clinic.

O/E lean, stoop-shouldered young man with rough unkempt hair, dirty clothes and reddish dry lips; 2 lymph nodes in the right anterior cervical triangle, 2 x 1.5 cm, tender, matted together and firm.

Investigations: (02/13/03) FNAC 'Granulomatous inflammation with necrosis suggestive of tuberculosis. Stain for AFB negative.'

Sputum smear/culture negative for AFB, Hb11 gm/dl, TLC-11000, P52, L20, E20, M08, ESR 32 mm.

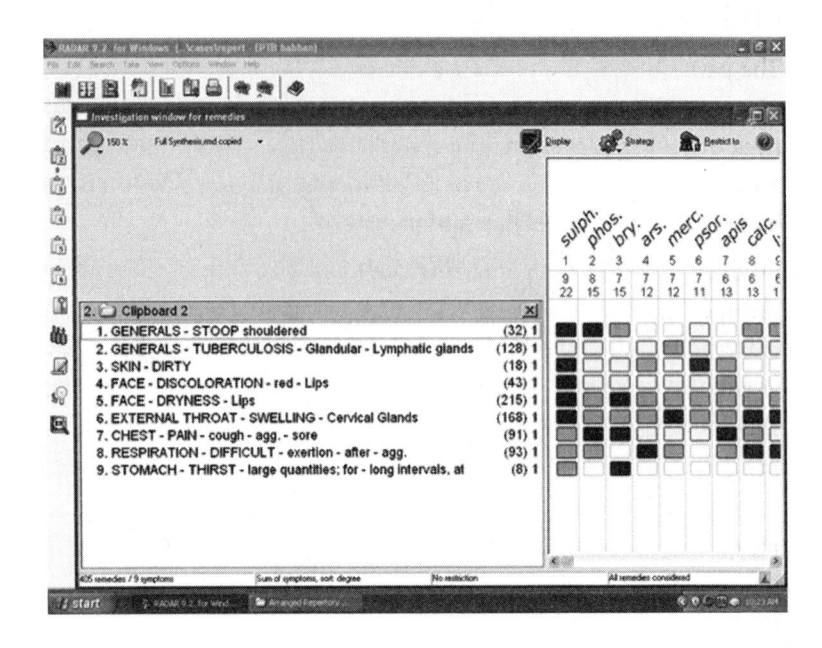

B was prescribed, on 01/30/03, *Sulph.* 30c x 1 dose every 15 days, *Tub.* 200c x 1 dose every 15 days, *Sil.* 6D tds every day. For acute coryza with fever *Ars. 30c* tds was used.

All the presenting symptoms gradually disappeared, 2 acute attacks of coryza and pain in chest were successfully treated with homeopathy. Lymph nodes became impalpable after 9 months. Investigations on 10/16/03: Hb 11.2gm/dl, TLC 5800, P50, L48, E01, M01, ESR 10 mm, chest X-ray (2747) 'right-sided thickened pleura, left hilum enlarged, no active lung lesion seen.' The weight of the patient was static at 48 kg.

Observation: Though the patient was cured of all the symptoms and the cervical lymph nodes had become impalpable, but the weight was static and the left hilum in X-ray chest was enlarged. Maybe he was not fully cured of the disease.

10. 03/06/03 to 06/05/03 and 09/30/04 to 11/15/04

MR, 24 yrs, M, Muslim from Bihar, low socio-economic strata, recently shifted to Delhi.

The patient came to the chest clinic on 03/06/03 for the treatment of cough with expectoration, chest pain and painful swellings in the neck of 3 weeks duration. The complaints started with fever lasting 4 days. The swellings in the neck were present before the fever but had recently become bigger and painful.

O/E tall, lean man with a narrow chest and pale face, liked being in the open air with friends, which he missed in the city. There were 2 enlarged lymph nodes in the right cervical region, 2 x 3 cm, matted together, tender and firm, with 3–4 small lymph nodes on both sides of the neck like a knotted cord.

Investigations: (03/06/03) chest X-ray (2835) 'pneumonitis in right paracardiac region'. Sputum smear/culture for AFB negative. FNAC. 'Granulomatous lesion with necrosis consistent with tuberculosis, no AFB seen', Hb11.5gm/dl, TLC 10,200, P49, L40, E05, M06, ESR 47 mm.

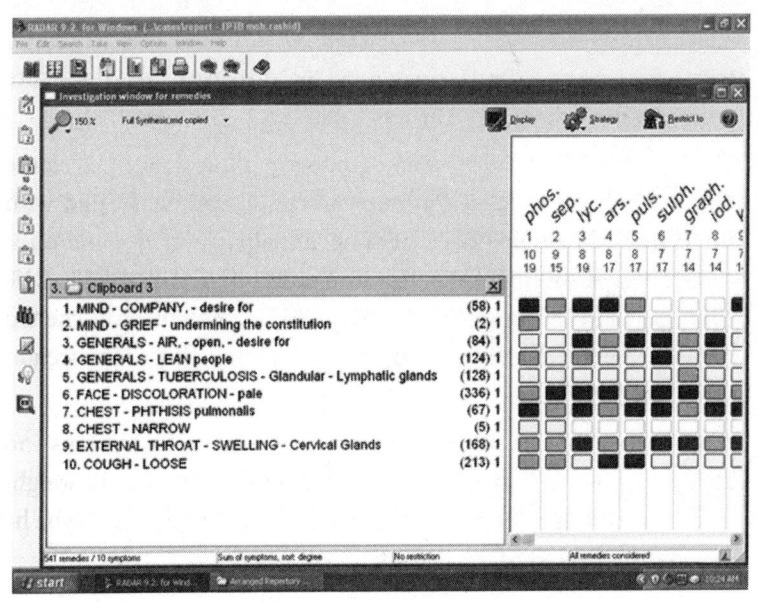

Phos. 30c x 1 dose once a week was given for 3 months from 03/06/03 to 06/05/03 with marked improvement in all the symptoms except in the size of the lymph nodes, chest X-ray (3828) 'bilateral hilar enlargement seen, aorta is unfolded.' The patch of pneumonitis in right para-cardiac region had resolved, Hb 12 gm/dl, TLC 5400, P 55, L 40, E 03, M 02, ESR 20 mm. *Sil. 6D* tds was added along with weekly *Phos. 30c* The patient went back to his village. He came back on 09/30/04 after about one year. The lymph node regressed initially, then became static, presently 1.5 cm, painless, discrete and mobile; *Tub. 200c* along with *Sil. 6D* tds and *Phos. 30c* x 1 dose once a week on 10/25/04 was given. After 6 weeks the lymph node had regressed to less than 0.5 cm in size. The patient went back to his village.

Observation: The grief of missing the open surrounding of his village was a contributory factor in the development of disease. Homeopathy acted simultaneously on mental as well as physical level. *Phos.* was effective in curing symptoms and pneumonitis, but had no effect on the size of lymph nodes. *Sil.* caused partial regression. Use of *Phos., Sil.* and *Tub.* simultaneously led to complete cure.

11. 04/17/03 to 10/17/03

K, 7 yrs, F, Hindu.

K was brought for homeopathic consultation by the mother on 04/17/03 for the complaints of painful swelling under the chin and cough for 2 months; cough more in the morning, with occasional vomiting and white expectoration; loss of weight; history of recurrent attacks of cold on exposure to cold air, yet liked being outdoors; poor eater.

O/E small-built, pale with rough, dry hair, 1 submental lymph node, 2x3 cm, tender, firm and mobile with multiple palpable lymph nodes, painless, less than 1 cm in size; enlarged uvula with sticky saliva.

Investigations: (04/10/03) Hb.-7.5 gm/dl, DLC P70, L20, E03, M01, ESR 40 mm; chest X-ray (1076) 'Hila are prominent with calcified foci.' FNAC (08/10/03) 'Granulomatous lesion with caseating necrosis compatible with TB, Stain for AFB positive'. Sputum smear/culture negative.

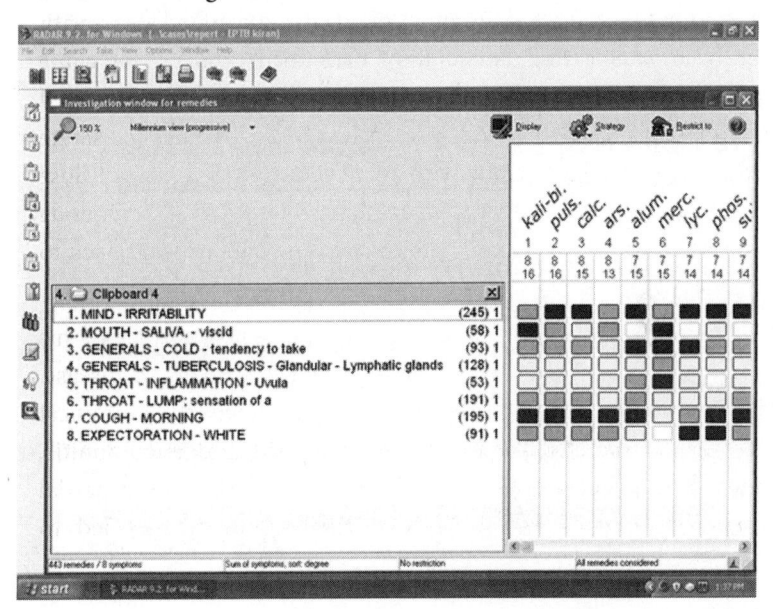

K was prescribed *Kali-bi. 30c* tds x 3 days, followed by *Sil. 6D* tds x 4 days a wk and *Tub. 200c* x 1 dose every 15 days for 1 month. The cough and expectoration was much reduced, treatment continued with *Tub. 200c* x 1 dose every 15 days and *Sil. 6D* tds for 5 months. 2 episodes of acute coryza were treated with *Puls. 30c*.

K was asymptomatic in 6 months and the lymph node reduced to 0.5 cm, soft in consistency, weight increase by 2 kg. Investigations (10/09/03) Hb 10.5 gm/dl, TLC 8500, P63, L33, E02, M02, ESR 24 mm; chest X-ray (3766) (11/06/03) 'lung fields clear, hila normal.'

Observation: This case reflected the importance of selection of constitutional remedy according to the presenting symptoms, along with the use of nosode and a leucocytic stimulant. An AFB positive patient was cured of TB with only homeopathy.

12. 06/12/03 to 12/14/03

KA, 37 yrs, F, Hindu, housewife.

KA came for homeopathic consultation on 06/12/03 for the treatment of a painful, gradually increasing swelling under the chin, noticed two months ago, pain in the epigastric region about an hour after eating, particularly after salads and loss of weight. History of PTB in husband one year ago.

O/E slightly obese (64 kg), very worried about her health, 2 submandibular lymph nodes, 2 x 3 cm, matted but not adherent to overlying skin.

Investigations: (06/12/03) Hb 12gm/dl, TLC 8,200, P72, L22, E04, M02, ESR 40 mm, chest X-ray (970) normal, FNAC 'Granulomatous lymphadenitis with necrosis consistent with TB, Stain for AFB negative.'

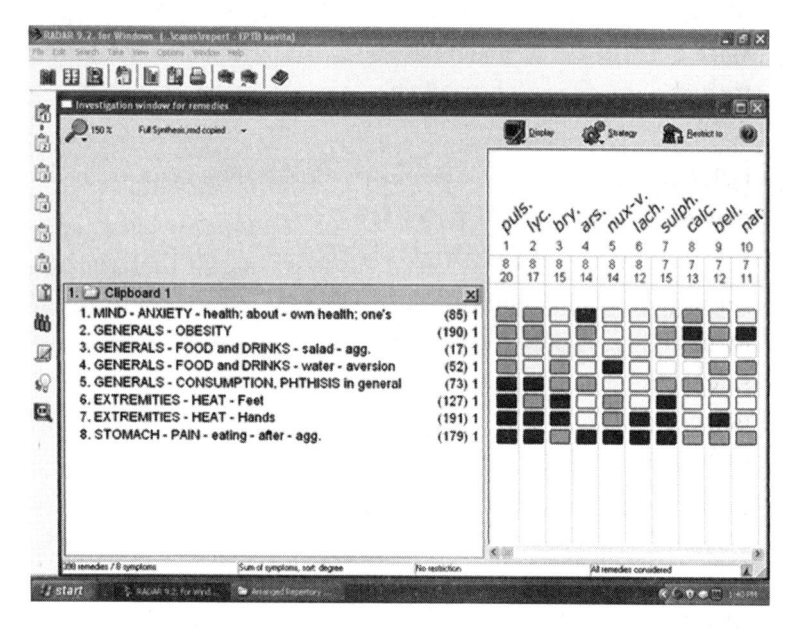

KA was prescribed *Puls. 30c* tds x 1 day in a wk, *Tub. 200c* x 1 dose once a wk and *Sil. 6D* tds.

The duration of treatment was 6 months with amelioration of gastric symptoms and pain, lymph nodes becoming impalpable. Haemogram on 11/06/03 showed Hb 13 gm/dl, TTLC 6,200, P66, L18, E04, M02, ESR 16 mm.

Observation: Patient was in the early stage of TB, which was effectively controlled by only homeopathy. Duration of treatment was shorter, as *Tub.* was used in weekly doses from the beginning.

13. 10/16/03 to 09/23/04

G, 9 yrs, M, Hindu, student.

G was brought by the mother on 10/16/03 for the homeopathic treatment of swellings in the neck of 1 year duration, associated with dry cough, more at night, on lying down, worse attack ended in vomiting; 3–4 episodes of epistaxis. History of recurrent attacks of cough with expectoration particularly at the change of season since 5 years, TB in maternal uncle. The worse attacks of cough treated with allopathic medicines, no history of treatment with ATT.

O/E small-built with pale anxious face; multiple enlarged, bilateral, painless, cervical lymph nodes like a knotted cord, one on right side matted, 2 x 2 cm, tender and adherent to overlying skin.

Investigations: (10/16/03) Hb 9.0 gm/dl, TLC 8,600, P44, L 46, E08, M 02, ESR 58 mm; chest X-ray 'Hilar prominence on the right side, lung fields clear.' FNAC 'granulomatous inflammation with necrosis consistent with TB, stain for AFB positive. Sputum smear/culture negative for AFB.

G was given *Dros. 30c* x 1 dose once in 15 days from 10/16/03 to 03/18/04. There was marked improvement in cough, but the lymph nodes were hardly reduced. *Sil. 6D* tds was added. The 2 medicines were given till 05/27/04, no cough and the lymph nodes further reduced. *Tub. 200c* x 1 dose in 15 days was added to previous 2 medicines. All the 3 medicines were given till 09/23/04.

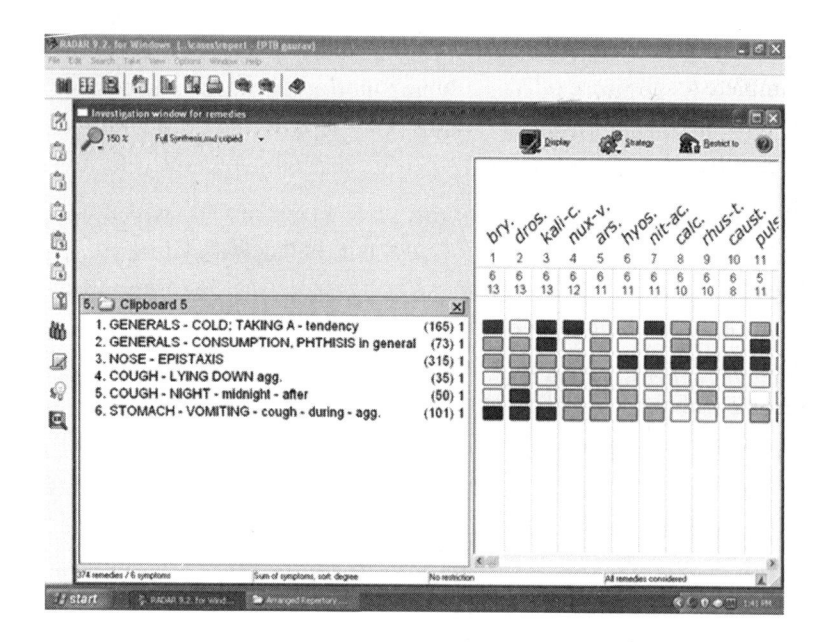

The total duration of treatment was 11 months leading to amelioration of all the symptoms and the lymph nodes became impalpable. Haemogram (09/23/04) Hb 11.5 gm/dl, TLC 7,200, P52, L38, E08, M02, ESR 26 mm.

Observation: This case reflected the role of each medicine in the cure of the disease. Complete reversal of pathology took place when constitutional medicine (patient-specific), disease-specific (nosode) and general stimulant medicines were given together.

14. 09/22/04 to 02/24/05

R, 20 yrs, M, medical student, Hindu.

R had suffered from PTB one year ago, treated with ATT Cat III for 6 months, well for 3 months, when a progressively increasing swelling was noticed on the right side of the neck along with weakness, feverishness and loss of appetite. FNAC confirmed it to be of tubercular pathology. He consulted his physician, who advised him to wait and watch the progress of the disease, as he had completed the course of ATT only 3 months ago. In the meantime he took *Sil.30c, 200c, Calc.-p. 30c, Baci. 200c, Tub. 200c* and *1M* one after other in single doses at two to three weeks interval without much effect.

O/E chest clinic (09/22/04) thin-built, fair, had acidity after eating fried food, itching after sweating and offensive sweat for 6 months; 1 lymph node in right anterior cervical triangle, painless, 2 x 2 cm, firm, mobile, not adherent to overlying skin; pitting on the nails of second and third right fingers.

Investigations: Hb 12.5 gm/dl, TLC 5,800, P46, L42, E08, M04, ESR 46 mm. Weight 62 kg. Chest X-ray 'old healed lesion in the right upper lung field.'

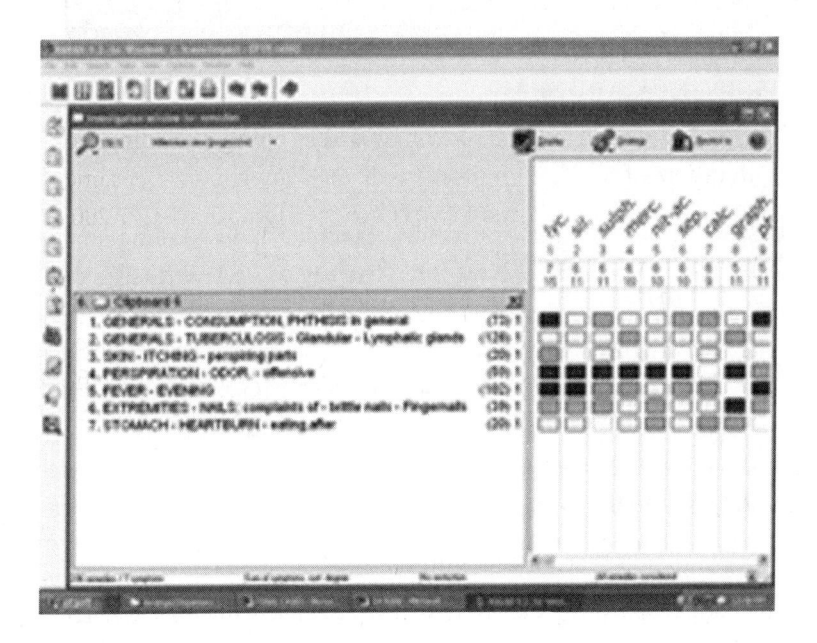

R was prescribed *Lyc. 200c* x 1 dose once a wk, *Tub. 1M* x one dose once in 15 days and *Sil. 6D* tds x 5 days a wk. (*Tub. 1M* was selected as he had it only a week ago).

R was monitored fortnightly. After a month the size of the lymph node started regressing, the offensive sweating reduced, the nails became better and appetite became normal. Treatment continued for five and a half months, when the lymph node was not palpable, the nails had become normal and he had gained in weight. Haemogram (02/24/05) Hb14.5/dl, TLC 5,400, P62, L30, E04, M04, ESR 20 mm.

Observation: Single doses of well selected medicine had no impact on the disease. Simultaneous use of medicines at three levels, constitutional, nosode and a stimulant to leucocytic activity brought about a sustained improvement in symptoms of the disease. With regular use, the improvement was noticed first in general well-being, then in symptoms followed by softening of lymph nodes at six weeks; finally the reduction in size.

15. 10/16/04 to 01/20/05

AS, 49 yrs, F, vice principal in school, Muslim from a well-to-do family.

AS complained of marked tiredness, lassitude and a swelling on the right side of neck since 6 months. History of recurrent colds and cough with yellow expectoration and occasional fever for last 2–3 yrs. She was extensively investigated at Holy Family Hospital for the cause of tiredness. FNAC (A04.465) (06/19/04) 'Granulomatous inflammation with necrosis suggestive of tuberculosis. Smear stained for acid fast bacillus is negative.'; Blood sugar fasting 96mg/dl and after 2 hrs. 107mg/dl; Thyroid stimulating hormone (TSH) 1.6μm/ml; Blood urea 14mg/dl, serum creatinine 0.6mg/dl, [Na+ 137, K+ 4.3, Cl- 101, HCO3 21] mEq/L, Total bilirubin 0.3 mg/dl, Total protein 7.4g/L, A/G ratio 1.2:1, SGPT(ALT) 28 u/l; SGOT(AST) 26 U/L, Alkaline phosphatase 124 IU/L; Hb 12.5 gm/dl, TLC 7200/cmm, P 70, L 28, Stabs 02, ESR 36 mm, platelets adequate and RBC normocytic; sputum for AFB negative; treated with Cat III ATT. The symptoms of fever and weight loss in the

Appendix: Case Histories of Tuberculosis

beginning of the disease improved with ATT, but there was no appreciable change in the size of the lymph nodes and tiredness.

O/E Chest clinic, fair, slightly plump with lax muscles, marked lassitude, symptoms out of proportion to the disease as shown by the investigations; 2 lymph nodes, 2 x 2 cm, painless, firm and mobile in right anterior cervical region; thyroid gland prominent, painless with a smooth surface.

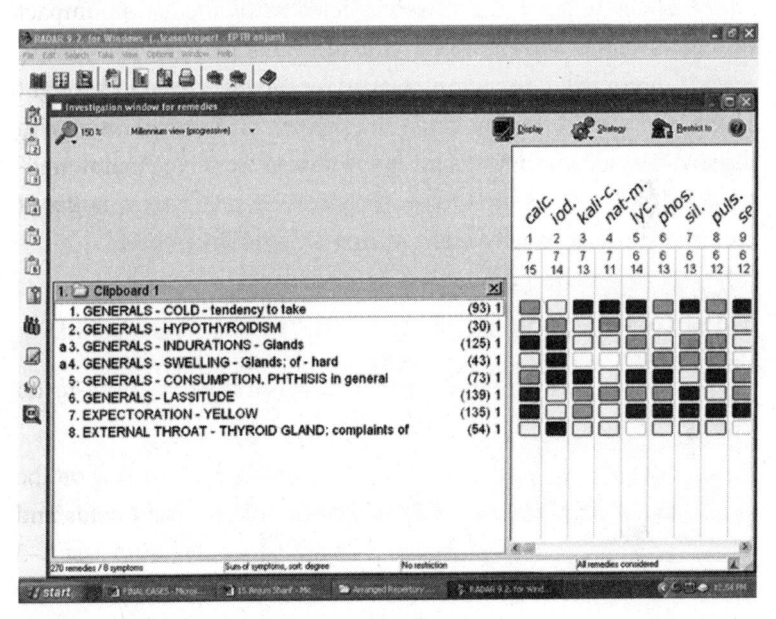

AS was prescribed on 10/16/04 *Calc-i. 30c* tds and *Tub. 1M* one dose every fortnight (this potency was selected as she had taken a dose only a week ago, as advised by another homeopath) for 3 months.

The symptoms of tiredness and lassitude showed immediate improvement. The swelling steadily reduced in size after a month. Patient felt well and swelling was not palpable after 3 months, Hb increased to 13.5 gm/dl, ESR reduced to 10 mm.

Observation: The persistent symptoms and feeling of sickness after a full course of ATT were effectively cured with homeopathic treatment.

16. 10/11/04 to 03/10/05

RSY, 35 yrs, M, Hindu, electrician in a government job.

RSY had the complaints of generalized weakness, loss of weight and enlargement of cervical lymph nodes since 1 year; chest X-ray and FNAC of the lymph node done in April 2004 revealed TB of lungs and lymph nodes, treated with Cat I ATT for six and a half months and *Phos. 30c* weekly doses for 2 months.

RSY was referred to the chest clinic on 10/11/04 for the painful cervical lymphadenopathy in spite of treatment, anxiety about his health and the fear that he might be suffering from some incurable disease like cancer, so it was futile to take any medicine and wanted to stop ATT. Since last 10 days he had fever coming on at 2 pm, chill at 4 pm, sweating at night, which brought down fever.

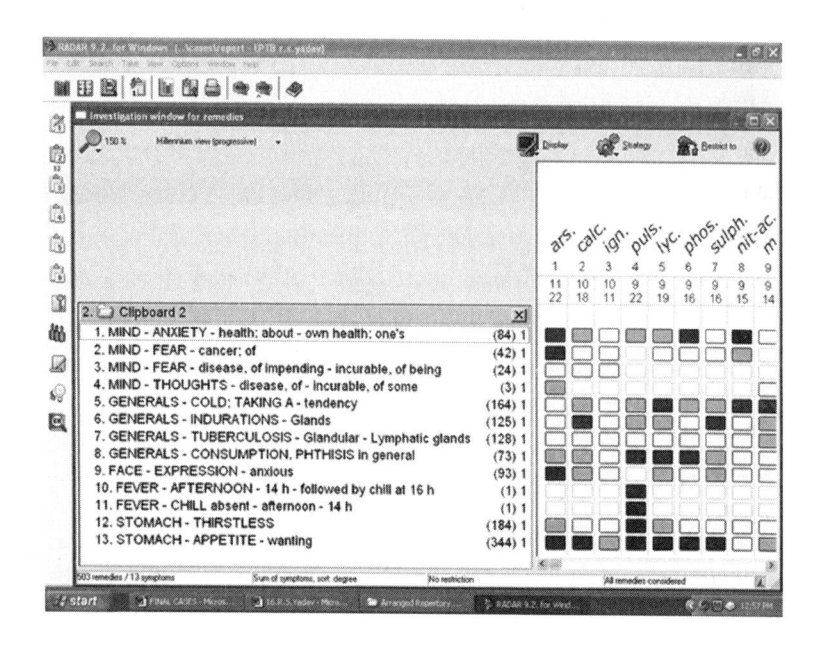

O/E lean, neatly dressed man with an anxious look, cold sensitive, had no appetite or thirst, whatever little he ate, remained a long time in the stomach and caused heartburn; multiple lymph nodes on the right side of the neck, 4–5 in the posterior cervical region, 2 were matted, 2 x 3 cm, tender firm, rest small, painless and discrete, a matted mass of 2–3 lymph nodes in the supraclavicular region, 5 x 2.5 cm, tender, cystic, adherent to overlying skin, no sinus formation.

Investigations: (10/11/04) Hb 10gm/dl, TLC 5,500, P46, L38, E11, M05, ESR 84 mm.

RSY was prescribed on 10/11/04. *Puls. 30c* tds for first week for fever, *Ars-i. 30c* tds and *Tub. 200c* once a week for next 2 weeks. After 3 weeks, there was no fever, and the anxiety was reduced. There after he was given *Tub. 200c* once a week, *Ars-i. 30c* tds once a week and *Sil. 6D* tds five days a week. *Puls. 30c* for fever/dyspepsia/frequent stools as required.

Size of the lymph nodes reduced steadily after six weeks. In less than three months lymph nodes were hardly palpable. Patient had completed nine months of ATT on 01/31/05, so it was stopped. Homeopathic treatment continued for next two months. Investigations (03/10/05): Hb13.0gm/dl, TLC 6,400, P56, L35, E06, M03, ESR 22 mm.

Follow-up: Patient has been followed till date, he has been well. He has been advised to take an occasional dose of *Tub. 1M* particularly after an episode of prolonged acute illness.

Observation: The cervical lymph nodes increased in size in spite of treatment of PTB and lymphadenopathy with conventional ATT and single doses of homeopathy. Selection of homeopathic constitutional medicine according to presenting complaints, simultaneous use of medicines targeting three levels of pathology and treatment of acute episodes with indicated homeopathic medicines led to steady recovery both at mental and physical planes.

17. 09/01/05 to 01/03/06

DK, 14 yrs, M, student, Hindu from low socio-economic strata.

DK had the following complaints for 3 years, insidiously increasing swelling in right thigh, painful on walking; attacks of cough with yellow, thick, easy and offensive expectoration, evening rise of fever, chest pain on inspiration and dyspnoea on exertion, weakness and loss of weight. He was investigated at All India Institute of Medical Sciences Hospital and referred to DOT centre of RNTCP on 08/31/05. Hb 9.5 gm/dl, TLC 9500, P 54, L 36, E 08, M O2, ESR 95 mm, FNAC (08/18/05) 'Aspirate from right inguinal swelling shows granulomatous inflammation with acid-fast bacilli, consistent with tuberculosis.' Chest X-ray normal; Sputum smear/ culture negative for AFB.

DK came to the homeopathic chest clinic on 09/01/2005 for symptomatic treatment as it was in the vicinity of the DOT centre. O/E inability to eat, no thirst, dryness of tongue, constipation, hard stool, gurgling sound in abdomen, generalized increased

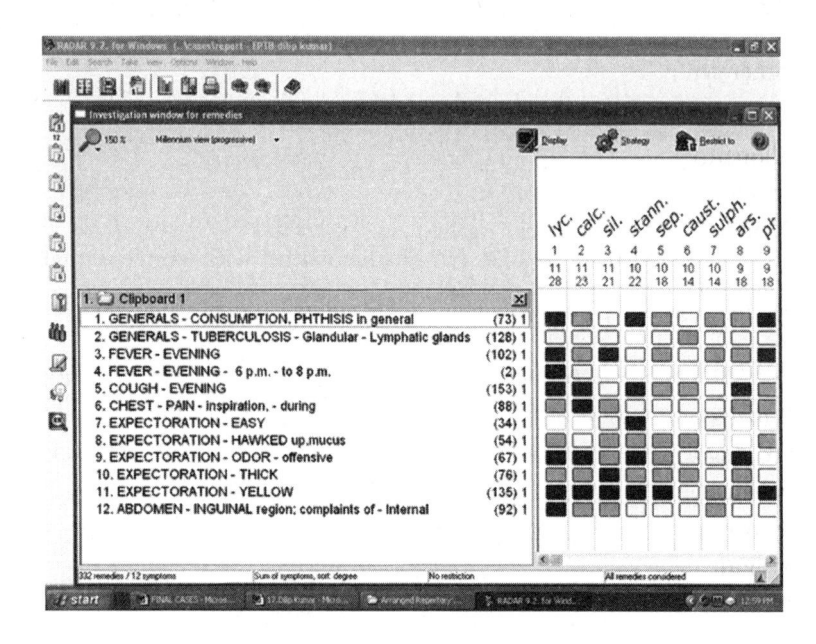

Appendix: Case Histories of Tuberculosis

sweat, especially on face and marked lassitude; tender, cystic, non-pulsating, swelling of matted inguinal glands, 8 cm x 8 cm.

DK was prescribed on 09/01/05 *Lyc. 200c* x 1 dose once a week and *Tub. 200c* x 1 dose once a wk. The cough, expectoration, fever and lassitude were first to improve, dyspnoea, chest pain and swelling started improving after 6 weeks. In between he had cough with white expectoration and wheezing of one week duration, treated with *Ars. 30c* twice a day x 1 week. The treatment continued till 01/03/06 when the patient also completed the ATT course of 6 months, after that he went to his village. Investigations (01/03/06) Hb 12.0gm/dl, TLC 6,200, P60, L32, E05, M05, ESR 25 mm.

DK was examined again on 07/10/06.The inguinal swelling was 4 x 3 cm, painless and mobile. He complained of dyspepsia (old symptoms) on empty stomach more in the evening and at night (10–11 pm). Repeat FNAC was positive for TB.

He was prescribed *Tub. 200c* x 1 dose a week, *Lyc. 200c* x 1 dose a week, *Sil. 6D* tds x 5 days a week.

The swelling was further reduced in size. Now 2 painless lymph nodes of 1.5 x 1.0 and 1.0 x 1.0 cm were palpable. There were no other symptoms. Treatment was continued for 2 more months.

Observation: The use of homeopathy (immune booster) along with allopathy (bactericidal) had a synergistic effect. Addition of *Sil. 6D* to *Tub. 200c* and *Lyc. 200c* further reduced the swelling to less than 1 cm x 1 cm and made the patient symptom-free.

18. 06/30/05 to 10/31/05

R, 42 yrs, F, Hindu housewife.

R had a prolonged attack of cough with expectoration two months ago, associated with loss of weight. She noticed gradually growing swellings in the neck three weeks ago; had severe backache, better by pressure; had a sensation of something sticking in the throat without expectoration. History of recurrent tonsillitis, cancer of breast in mother.

O/E sickly with a suffering expression, chilly, sensitive to draught of air, had desire for lime; enlarged lymph nodes, one behind the ear and a chain of nodes in the right anterior cervical region, 1 x 3 cm, tender, matted but not adherent to the overlying skin.

Investigations: (06/30/05) chest X-ray 'old healed lesion in right mid-zone suggestive of TB'; FNAC 'caseating material with superimposed acute infection, stain for AFB positive'; Sputum smear/culture negative for AFB; Hb 11.5 gm/dl, TLC 12,500, P60, L28, E10, M02, ESR 76 mm.

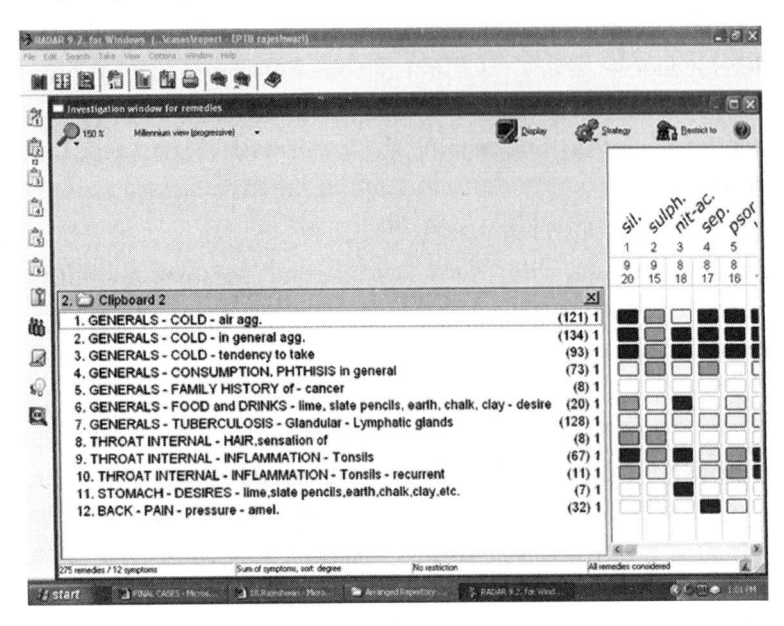

R was prescribed: *Sil.* 30c x 3 doses once a week, *Tub.* 200c x 1 dose once a week and *Sil.* 6D tds x 5 days a week; on 06/30/05,.

The patient was symptom-free, lymph nodes not palpable in four months and she gained weight by 4 kg. Haemogram on 10/31/05: Hb 13gm/dl, TLC 6,500, P65, L25, E06, M04, ESR 26 mm.

Observation: AFB positive lymphadenopathy was cured with only homeopathy in four months. *Sil.* was used in higher potency as a constitutional medicine and in lower potency (6D) as a general stimulant with beneficial results.

Appendix: Case Histories of Tuberculosis

19. 09/08/05 to 12/12/05

V, 11 yrs, M, Hindu, student.

V was brought by the father on 09/08/05 for the treatment of the complaints of fever for 1 week and pain in the back for 2 weeks. The father had a successful homeopathic treatment of TB lymphadenitis six months ago and was visiting the clinic for a follow-up.

V had pain in the lumbar region of the back, less in the morning, maximum in the evening, associated with lot of weakness, lassitude; developed fever after 1 week, hot at 2 pm, followed by chill at 4 pm and sweating at night; no thirst, poor eater; irritable, obstinate and wept easily; losing weight. History of recurrent gastroenteritis; TB in father.

Investigations: (09/08/05) Hb 11.70 gm/dl, TLC 11,600, P69, L25, E06, ESR 18 mm, chest X-ray 'left hilar and paratracheal lymph nodes enlarged, no active lung lesion seen. X-ray of the lumbar spine normal.

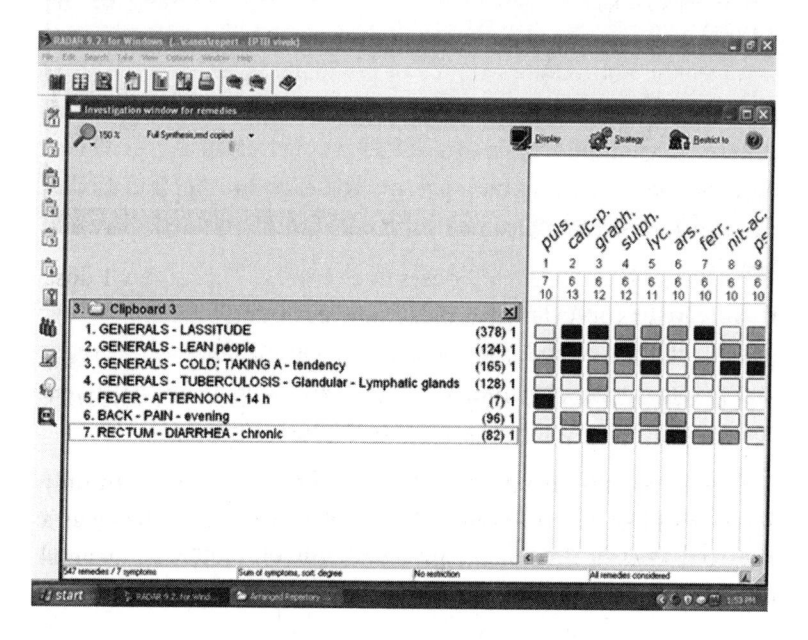

1. GENERALS - LASSITUDE	(378)	1
2. GENERALS - LEAN people	(124)	1
3. GENERALS - COLD; TAKING A - tendency	(165)	1
4. GENERALS - TUBERCULOSIS - Glandular - Lymphatic glands	(128)	1
5. FEVER - AFTERNOON - 14 h	(7)	1
6. BACK - PAIN - evening	(96)	1
7. RECTUM - DIARRHEA - chronic	(82)	1

Remedies: puls. / calc-p. / graph. / sulph. / lyc. / ars. / ferr. / nit-ac. / ps.

V was treated with *Puls*. *30c* tds for the first week, followed by once a week and further on as required basis; *Calc-p. 6D* tds and *Tub. 200c* once a week. Occasional episode of nausea with vomiting in the beginning treated with *Ip. 30c*; he was asymptomatic after one month with occasional bouts of fever controlled by *Puls. 30c*. The duration of treatment was three months, chest X-ray (12/12/05) 'normal, no enlargement of hilar and paratracheal lymph nodes'; Hb 12.5gm/dl, TLC 7,400, P62, L34, E03, M01, ESR 08 mm, weight gain of 4 kg.

Follow-up: The patient has been asymptomatic and healthy till date.

Observation: Patient was a case of incipient TB lymphadenopathy cured rapidly with homeopathy and maybe the development of spinal TB was thwarted.

20. 11/16/05 to 02/22/06

P, 20 yrs, F, Hindu, married.

P had delivered a female child one and a half years ago through normal delivery. She was depressed, had no appetite or thirst, after two months noticed appearance of gradually increasing swellings in the neck, feverishness in the evening and loss of weight; husband suffered from multidrug-resistant PTB, being treated at a TB centre near the chest clinic; his both parents and elder brother had died of TB. Her own brother also had suffered from TB, treated, alive and healthy.

P came to the chest clinic for the treatment of swellings in the neck, pain in the lower abdomen worse on bending forward, at night and before menses; felt like weeping all the time for no particular reason, especially at night and before menses.

O/E anaemic with a sickly anxious face, desire for sweets and hot tea at frequent intervals, frightful dreams of dead persons; three enlarged anterior cervical lymph nodes, one on right side 3 x 3 cm and two on left side 2 x 2 cm, tender, matted, not fixed to skin.

FNAC (No. 57/05) 10/09/2005 'Tubercular Lymphadenitis, no AFB seen'; chest X-ray 'bilateral prominence of hilar regions, lung fields normal'; Hb 8.5 gm/dl, TLC 9,200, P55, L35, E06, M04, ESR 84 mm.

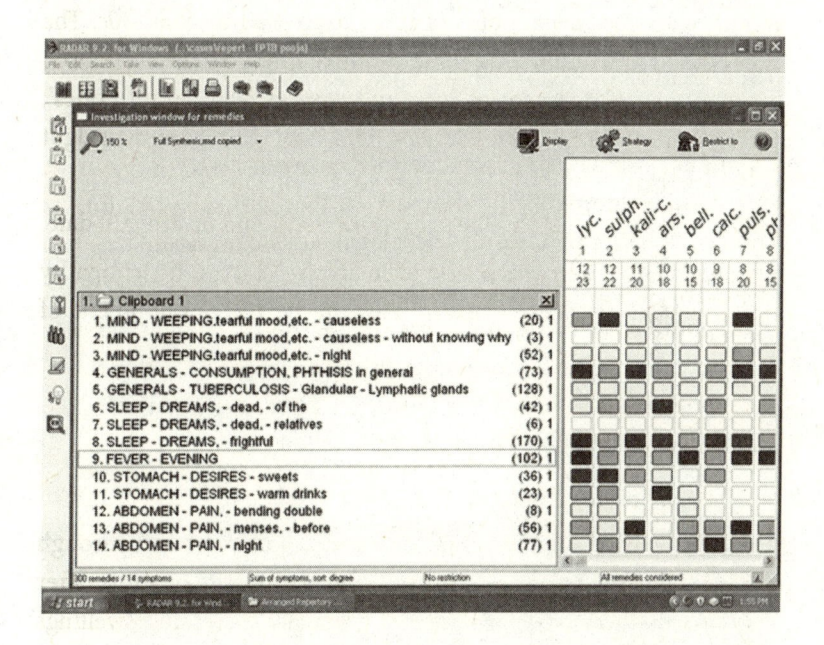

[Screenshot of RADAR 9.2 for Windows repertorization showing the following rubrics:]

#	Rubric	Count
1	MIND - WEEPING,tearful mood,etc. - causeless	(20) 1
2	MIND - WEEPING,tearful mood,etc. - causeless - without knowing why	(3) 1
3	MIND - WEEPING,tearful mood,etc. - night	(52) 1
4	GENERALS - CONSUMPTION, PHTHISIS in general	(73) 1
5	GENERALS - TUBERCULOSIS - Glandular - Lymphatic glands	(128) 1
6	SLEEP - DREAMS, - dead, - of the	(42) 1
7	SLEEP - DREAMS, - dead, - relatives	(6) 1
8	SLEEP - DREAMS, - frightful	(170) 1
9	FEVER - EVENING	(102) 1
10	STOMACH - DESIRES - sweets	(36) 1
11	STOMACH - DESIRES - warm drinks	(23) 1
12	ABDOMEN - PAIN, - bending double	(8) 1
13	ABDOMEN - PAIN, - menses, - before	(56) 1
14	ABDOMEN - PAIN, - night	(77) 1

Top remedies: lyc, sulph, kali-c, ars, bell, calc, puls, pt

She was prescribed *Lyc.* 0/1 in LM potency to be taken three times a day and *Tub. 200c* as a weekly dose till 02/22/06. There was steady improvement in all her complaints and reduction in the size of lymph nodes to 0.5–1.0 cm, painless, soft and discrete; Hb 11.5 gm/dl, TLC 6,500, P65, L25, E05, M05, ESR 26 mm, weight gain of 3 kg.

Observation: LM potency was used to avoid any medicinal aggravation as it was felt that frequent repetition of *Lyc.* would be beneficial.

21. 02/12/05 to 05/10/05

P, 31 yrs, F, Hindu, married, living separately from husband since 5 yrs.

P had suffered from AFB positive, tubercular abscess, in the right neck one year ago treated with Cat II ATT for 8 months, from 04/08/05 to 12/02/05. The abscess had healed, but 2 enlarged lymph nodes remained; had lot of anxiety about her and her son's health.

P came for homeopathic treatment of enlarged nodes in the neck with pain extending to the shoulder on the right side; pain in the lower back better by pressure, sleeplessness, weakness and hair fall.

O/E thin, emaciated with anxious look, restlessness at about midnight, fear of being alone, two lymph nodes in right anterior cervical region, 2 x 2 cm, tender, discrete, firm and adherent to underlying tissue. Chest X-ray (3079) on 12/08/05 normal, Hb 10.5 gm/dl, TLC 7,800, P46, L42, E04, M08, ESR 42 mm.

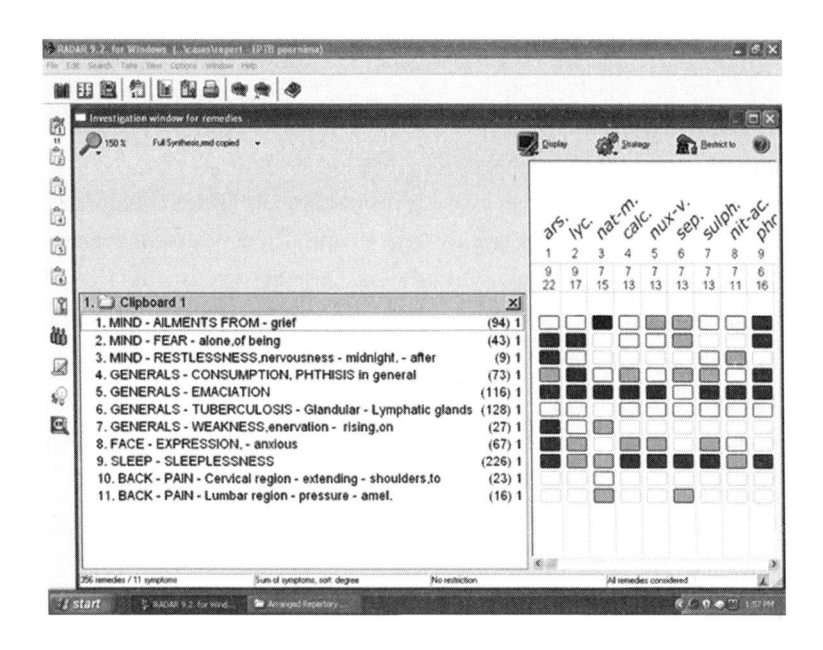

P was prescribed *Ars. 200c* once a week, *Tub. 200c* once a week and *Sil. 6D* tds for first three weeks as anxiety was the prominent presentation, followed by *Nat-m. 200c* once a week, *Tub. 200c* once a week and *Sil. 6D* tds till three months when she had no symptoms and lymph nodes were soft, less than 1 cm in size. Investigations (05/10/05) Hb 12.5gm/dl, TLC 6,600, P 58, L 32, E 04, M 06, ESR 18 mm.

Follow-up: P attended the clinic for next 4 months, treated for hair fall with Arnica Hair Oil and Shampoo, one acute attack of hoarseness and pain in throat with *Phos. 200c* followed by a dose of *Tub. 200c*.

Observation: ATT had healed the abscess, but the patient still felt sick with anxiety, weakness and enlarged lymph nodes. Homeopathic treatment made her asymptomatic and the lymph nodes regressed.

22. 02/15/05 to 06/08/05

C, 35 yrs, F, Hindu, married.

C came to the chest clinic for the treatment of swellings in the neck of seven months' duration; had given birth to a third female child about a year ago, which was not received well by the family and had caused depression in her. The swelling first appeared on the left side, treated at a hospital after investigations with ATT, took it for 1 month with reduction in the size of the swelling, went to her village and stopped the treatment. After two months another similar swelling appeared on the right side and she was losing weight. C did not go back to the hospital for fear of being scolded, so came for homeopathic consultation on 02/15/05.

O/E untidy appearance, cheerful and haughty, fond of highly seasoned food, very thirsty, drank water often in large quantities at a time; felt burning sensation in hands and feet, had profuse, offensive perspiration at night, felt worse after a bath so did not like a bath. Two large lymph nodes one on each side, painless, 3 x 4 cm, firm, discrete and mobile. Investigations (02/15/05) FNAC 'Tuberculous Lymphadenitis'. Chest X-ray normal, Hb 10.4 gm/dl, TLC 7, 800, P57, L40, E03, ESR 54 mm.

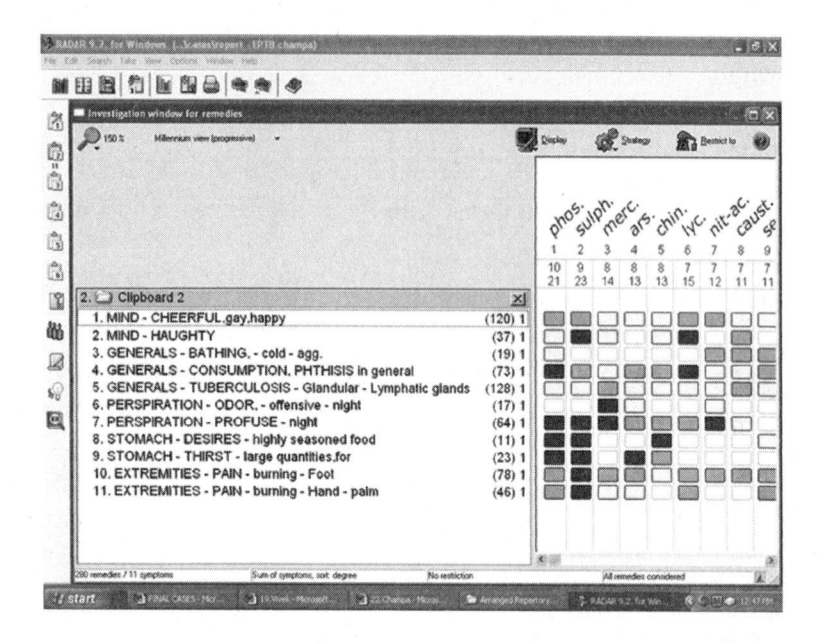

She was prescribed *Sulph. 30c* once a week, *Sil. 6D* tds and *Tub. 200c* once a week.

After 4 months lymph nodes decreased to less than 1 cm, became soft. Hb 12.8 gm/dl, TLC 5,600, P 65, L30, E03, M02, ESR 24 mm; increase in weight by 3 kg.

Observation: Mental trauma from family's reaction to the birth of third female child led to the development of TB lymphadenitis, single constitutional medicine along with nosode and general stimulant cured the patient totally of mental and physical disease.

23. 02/24/05 to 06/16/05

K, 25 yrs, M, Muslim, tailor from very low socio-economic strata.

K had TB cervical lymphadenopathy of three years' duration, treated with Cat III ATT for 8 months, the size of lymph nodes became static after initial decrease with no improvement in the symptoms; complained of pain in the neck, more during winter and on taking cold drinks; frequent attacks of sore throat always started from right side. His maternal aunt, living with him, suffered from PTB. FNAC done on 01/01/05 (after ATT), at a big hospital (Safdarjung Hospital, New Delhi) of the city reported, 'Smear from nodule in the right posterior cervical region reveals caseating tuberculous lymphadenitis, stain for AFB positive.'

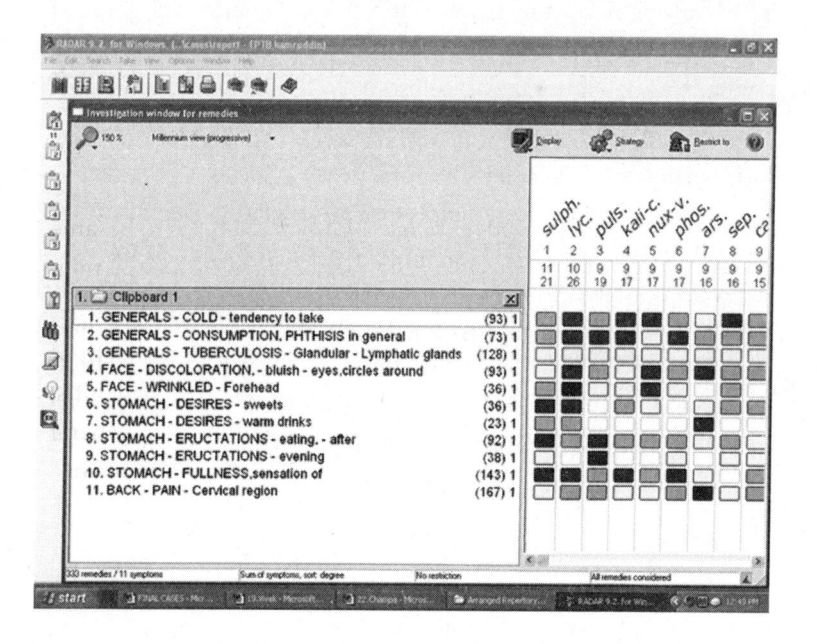

K came for homeopathic consultation on 02/24/05. O/E sickly yellow complexion, bluish circle around eyes, vertical furrow on the forehead and greying of hair; preferred and felt better with hot food and warm drinks, desired sweets, little food made him full, flatulent after food and in the evenings; multiple lymph nodes in the right posterior cervical region, 1–2 x 2 cm, painful, firm, discrete and mobile. Chest X-ray normal, Hb 9.6 m/dl, TLC 6,600, P50, L42, E06, M02, ESR 46 mm.

K was prescribed *Lyc. 30c* once a week, *Tub. 200c* once a week and *Sil. 6D* tds x five days a week; on 02/24/05. *Lyc. 30c* changed to *200c* after three months when improvement had become static.

At the end of four months, the patient was asymptomatic, lymph nodes not palpable, had gained weight by 2 kg, Hb 12.6 gm/dl, TLC 5,800, P 60, L32, E04, M04, ESR 18 mm.

Observation: Eight months of ATT had no effect on the disease or on the symptoms, may be due to multidrug-resistance while four months of homeopathic treatment made patient symptom-free, and the lymph nodes became impalpable.

24. 01/02/06 to 04/17/06

S, M, 9 yrs, student in primary school, Hindu.

S was brought by the parents for the complaints of gradually increasing swelling in the neck, fever in the evening associated with cough, scanty white expectoration, once streaked with blood, and weight loss of three months' duration.

O/E small-built, weak, anaemic with easy flushing of the face on exertion, pain in the chest aggravated on coughing, deep breathing and physical exertion; 2–3 lymph nodes on each side of the neck, 0.5–2.0 cm, painless, firm and mobile, axillary lymph nodes also enlarged on both sides. Investigations (01/02/ 06) Hb.-9.8gm/dl, TLC 7,600, P56, L27, E08, M09, ESR 28 mm, chest X-ray 'left hilum prominent, right costophrenic angle blunted.' FNAC 'Reactive granulomatous inflammation consistent with TB, no AFB seen.' Sputum smear/culture negative for AFB.

Appendix: Case Histories of Tuberculosis

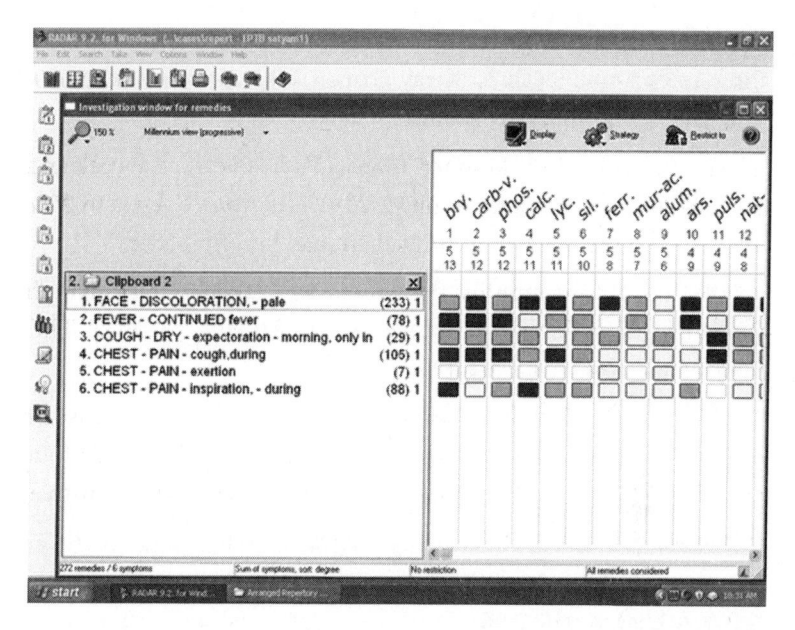

S was treated with *Bry. 30c* tds for 1 week, *Ferr-p. 6D* tds for 3 weeks, no pain in chest and fever after one month but the lymph nodes were same. He was prescribed *Tub. 200c* x once a week and *Sil. 6D* tds x six a week.

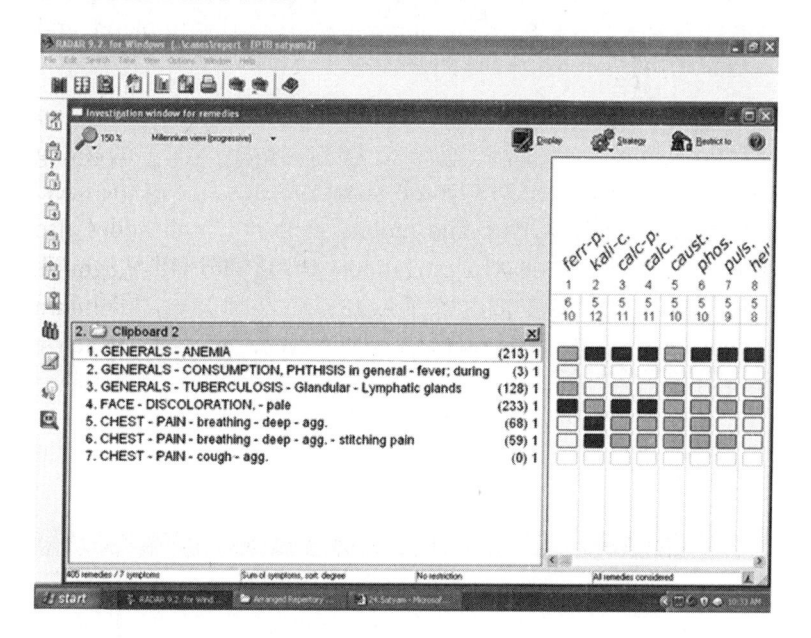

He was asymptomatic on 04/17/06, chest X-ray 'Bronchovascular markings prominent in bilateral upper lobes, costophrenic angles clear', Hb 14.1 gm/dl, TLC 5,800, P 48, L 42, E 06, M 04, ESR 9 mm.

Observation: An early case of early TB effectively treated with homeopathy in three and a half months. *Fer-p.* treated the anaemia, pain in chest and fever.

Follow-up: Patient continued to attend the clinic for one year, there was no recurrence.

25. 08/05/06 to 11/13/06

P, 5 yrs, M, Hindu, adopted child.

P was brought for homeopathic consultation by the mother who had noticed gradually increasing swellings in his neck for three months; he did not feel hungry (ask for food), but when made to eat a little, appetite returned, had a great liking for hot milk, sweated profusely especially on the head while sleeping; history of recurrent attacks of cold since childhood.

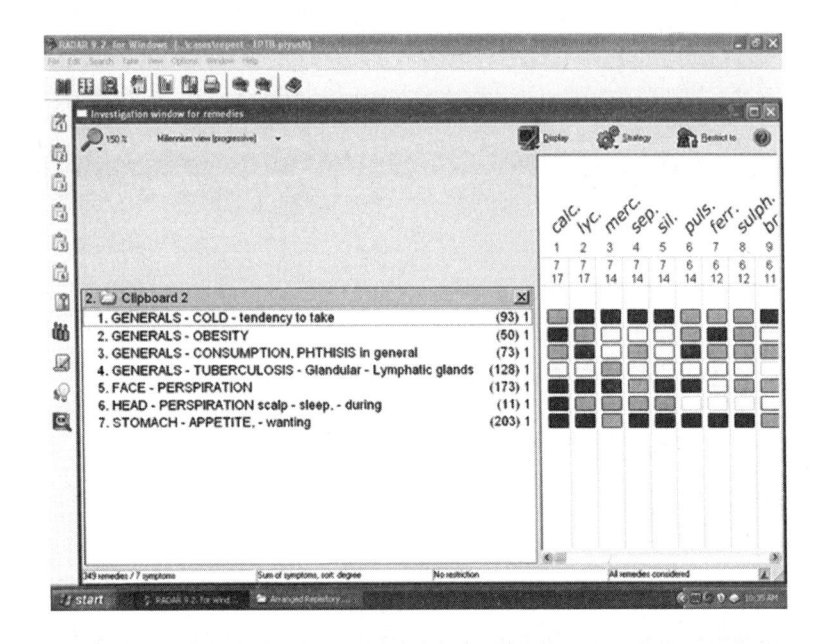

Appendix: Case Histories of Tuberculosis 211

O/E fair, flabby child with a sweaty face, multiple bilateral lymph nodes in the anterior cervical region, painless discrete, 0.5 x 2.0 cm, like a knotted cord, chest X-ray (07/21/06) normal, FNAC 'granulomatous lesion with caseation, no AFB seen.' Hb 9.2 gm/dl, TLC 7200, DLC P63, L31, E06, ESR 38 mm.

On 08/05/16, he was prescribed *Calc. 30c*, 1 dose once a week, *Tub. 200c*, 1 dose once a week and *Sil. 6D* tds till 11/13/06.

P did not have any attack of cold during 3 months, sweating reduced, asked for food and lymph nodes became impalpable. Hb 11.0 gm/dl, TLC 6,400, P55, L40, E03, M02, ESR 11 mm, weight gain of 2 kg.

Observation: The respiratory allergy, anorexia and tubercular lymphadenopathy were cured with regular use of single constitutional medicine in the regime along with nosode and general stimulant.

References

Anesi, J. 'Infection Control & Hospital Epidemiology', journal of *The Society for Healthcare Epidemiology of America*. https://www.eurekalert.org/pub_releases/2018-10/sfheari103018.php October 30, 2018.

Bellavite, P., Ortolani, R., Pontarollo, F., Piasere, V., Benato, G., Conforti, A. 'Immunology and Homeopathy. 5. The Rationale of the "*Simile*"', *Oxford Journals, Evidence-based Complementary and Alternative Medicine*, June, 2007; 4 (2): 149-63.

Chand, K.S. 'Homeopathy in the Treatment of Tuberculosis', *American Journal of Homeopathic Medicine*, Summer, 2013, vol. 102, no. 2.

Chand, K.S., Kapoor, P. 'Case reports on integrated management of tubercular disease', *Homeopathy*, 2017, 106 (2): 214-22.

Chand, K.S., Manchanda, R.K., Mittal, R., Batra, S., Banavaliker, J.N., De, I. 'Homeopathic treatment in addition to standard care in multi drug resistant pulmonary tuberculosis: A randomized, double blind, placebo controlled clinical trial', *Homeopathy*, 2014, 103: 97-107.

Chand, Kusum S., Kapoor, P. 'Two Case Reports of Integrated Management of Antibiotic Resistant Urinary Tract Infection', *Homeopathy*, 2020, 109 (02): 92-106.

Chand, S.K., Manchanda, R.K., Batra, S., Mittal, R. 'Homeopathy in the Treatment of Tubercular Lymphadenitis (TBLN): An Indian Experience', *Homeopathy*, 2011, 100 (3): 157-67.

Deretic, V., Delgado, M., Vergne, I., et al. 'Autophagy in Immunity Against *Mycobacterium tuberculosis*: a Model System to Dissect Immunological Roles of Autophagy', *Current Topics in Microbiology and Immunology*, 2009, 335: 169–88.

Danninger, T., Gallenberger, K., Kraeling, J. 'Immunologic changes in healthy probands and HIV infected patients after oral administration of *Staphylococcus aureus 12C*: a pilot study', *British Homeopathic Journal*, 2000, 89 (3): 106–15.

Studd, J., Seang, L.T., Chervenak, F.A. (eds). *Current Progress in Obstetrics and Gynaecology*, vol. 2, Suketu P. Kothari: Tree Life Media, Mumbai, India, 2014, pp. 319–36.

World Health Organization (WHO). 'High levels of antibiotic resistance found worldwide, new data shows', *Media Centre*, News releases, 2018.

Wynn, S.G. 'Studies on use of homeopathy in animals', *Journal of the American Veterinary Medical Association (USA)*, 1998, (5) 212: 719–24.